'*Queering Gestalt Therapy* is a truly pertinent and seminal contribution to the field of psychotherapy, irrespective of therapeutic orientation and training. This volume offers readers a breadth of understanding in its leading-edge discussion of the complexities and nuances in considering gender identities, sexual orientations, and relationship diversities. Readers will be rewarded with an essential broadening of awareness-informing-understanding, perspective, and clinical practice across the human landscape.'

Allan Singer, *Psychotherapist in Private Practice, Boston, MA, USA*

'Thanks to all who contributed to this timely anthology. I was simultaneously enlivened and brought up to date on reading through the diverse voices of contributors. This book makes an important and belated addition to our gestalt field. Anyone practising gestalt therapy with a general population today needs to read it.'

Malcolm Parlett PhD, *Author of* Future Sense, *former editor of the British Gestalt Journal*

Queering Gestalt Therapy

The first peer-reviewed book of its kind, this important volume addresses a current gap in the field of gestalt therapy: that the practice—and psychotherapy more broadly—still suffers from pervasive hetero- and cis-normativity.

This book offers gestalt-therapy-based research and training material on gender, sex, and relationship diversity (GSRD), including chapters on a variety of GSRD issues and how therapists can become more GSRD-sensitive. The contributors position themselves across the whole spectrum of GSRD and offer their voices as an invitation to further queer the gestalt community with diverse content ranging from academic, research-oriented pieces to experiential, reflective perspectives. Featured chapters explore topics including gender-radical clients, sex and sexuality, relationship diversity, integrating GSRD and gestalt therapy, and addressing heteronormativity in gestalt therapy training.

Queering Gestalt Therapy is for everyone who is interested in gender, sex, and relationship diversity, especially as they relate to gestalt therapy practice. This book will be especially useful for therapists, supervisors, coaches, and students of gestalt therapy.

Ayhan Alman is a queer psychotherapist with a Muslim, Middle Eastern context, and western upbringing. He trained as a gestalt psychotherapist at Metanoia Institute in London. Therapeutically, he is interested in how prejudice and bias impacts on the mental health of marginalised communities.

John Gillespie is a gestalt therapist based in London. He is a founding director of New Gestalt Voices and longstanding editor of the *NGV International Journal*. He works as a freelance consultant in the charity/public sectors, combining this with low cost therapy work.

Vikram Kolmannskog, Dr.Philos., is a queer-of-colour professor, gestalt therapist, and writer. He trained at, and currently works as a professor at, the Norwegian Gestalt Institute. In addition, he has a private therapy and supervision practice near Oslo and offers training both nationally and internationally. He is the author of several books, including *The Empty Chair: Tales from Gestalt Therapy* (Routledge, 2018).

Queering Gestalt Therapy

An Anthology on Gender, Sex & Relationship Diversity in Psychotherapy

Edited by Ayhan Alman, John Gillespie and Vikram Kolmannskog

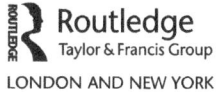
Routledge
Taylor & Francis Group

LONDON AND NEW YORK

Designed cover image: © adike/Shutterstock

First published 2023
by Routledge
4 Park Square, Milton Park, Abingdon, Oxon OX14 4RN

and by Routledge
605 Third Avenue, New York, NY 10158

*Routledge is an imprint of the Taylor & Francis Group,
an informa business*

British Library Cataloguing-in-Publication Data
A catalogue record for this book is available from the British Library

Library of Congress Cataloging-in-Publication Data
Names: Alman, Ayhan, editor. | Gillespie, John (Psychotherapist), editor. |
Kolmannskog, Vikram, editor.
Title: Queering gestalt therapy : an anthology on gender, sex &
relationship diversity in psychotherapy / edited by Ayhan Alman, John
Gillespie and Vikram Kolmannskog.
Description: Abingdon, Oxon ; New York, NY : Routledge, 2023. | Includes
bibliographical references and index.
Identifiers: LCCN 2022047724 (print) | LCCN 2022047725 (ebook) | ISBN
9781032371092 (paperback) | ISBN 9781032371108 (hardback) | ISBN
9781003335344 (ebook)
Subjects: LCSH: Gestalt therapy--Case studies. | Sexual
minorities--Psychology. | Sexual minorities--Mental health.
Classification: LCC RC489.G4 Q44 2023 (print) | LCC RC489.G4 (ebook) |
DDC 616.89/143--dc23/eng/20221223
LC record available at https://lccn.loc.gov/2022047724
LC ebook record available at https://lccn.loc.gov/2022047725

ISBN: 978-1-032-37110-8 (hbk)
ISBN: 978-1-032-37109-2 (pbk)
ISBN: 978-1-003-33534-4 (ebk)

DOI: 10.4324/9781003335344

Typeset in Times New Roman
by SPi Technologies India Pvt Ltd (Straive)

Contents

Acknowledgements

This project has been longstanding, and we have leant on a lot of others in the making of it. We want particularly to thank those who contributed peer reviews and whose support was instrumental in getting the chapters to the high standard they are. We acknowledge thus the support from Dr Bernadette Latuch, Schrusch, Dr Kamila Bialy, Dr Rhys Price-Robertson, Dr Melissa Sedmak, Chris O'Malley, Dr Adam Kincel, Koyote Millar, Dr Saya Karavadra, Steve Ausbury, and Andrés Lekanger (Chemfriendly Norge).

We want to thank New Gestalt Voices for providing a home and platform for developing the book and soliciting initial contributions.

The GSD special interest group of IAAGT (The International Association for the Advancement of Gestalt Therapy) particularly co-chairs Dr Daniel Bak and Billy Desmond were incredibly supportive of the project in the early days – they believed in us, and the group helped shape this from seed of an idea into the full-grown book it is today.

Likewise, we owe thanks to Dr Leanne O'Shea for her early encouragement and offers to support the development of this project.

And we would like to thank Dominic Davies of Pink Therapy for providing additional contexts around GSRD terminology and its evolution, as well as Dr Alex Iantaffi – one of the co-authors of 'Life isn't binary' – for their support with GSRD theory.

There are many more people and organisations in the psychotherapy field like Pink Therapy, to whom we owe credit for having innovated around GSRD issues, and without whom this book would undoubtedly not have taken the shape and form it has. We owe debts of gratitude to all who have led with their own truths and vulnerability in educating us as authors and the wider psychotherapy field in how to work with GSRD clients.

Additionally, we each have drawn on our own personal supports that have held us above water in those moments when aspects of our queer identities have not been supported elsewhere in the psychotherapy world.

I (John) particularly wish to thank members of my supervision group at 'London Friend' – Keith Barber, Sarah Reilly, Alec Scott Rook, and Hillary Ratnasabapathy for the love and support they consistently gave me. Likewise, I want to thank fellow editors Vikram and Ayhan for their support.

I (Ayhan) thank my fellow editors Vikram and John for their unbound support and care throughout the editing process and beyond. I thank my teachers and trainers from Metanoia Institute, Relational Change, and the Contemporary Institute for Clinical Sexology (CICS) who were instrumental in developing my psychotherapy practice. And I thank my loved ones and friends who offered a nourishing ground in times of stress.

I (Vikram) thank my fellow editors John and Ayhan. I have enjoyed working together on this book with you. As a queer gestalt therapist I have also felt supported and inspired by the GSD special interest group of IAAGT, in particular the smaller group of LGBTQ psychotherapists meeting regularly under that umbrella. I am grateful to each individual member as well as the group as a whole. Finally, I thank my colleagues at the Norwegian Gestalt Institute for support and encouragement, generally as well as specifically when it comes to my GSRD work.

We wish to thank Margaret Brady (Chair of Editorial Board) from *Inside Out Journal: The Irish Journal for Humanistic and Integrative Psychotherapists* for giving permission to republish Billy Desmond's piece and Gro Skottun, editor of Norsk Gestalttidsskrift, for giving permission to republish Vikram Kolmannskog's piece.

Finally, we thank Dr Lynne Jacobs for her support and acknowledgment with her foreword.

Foreword

Lynne Jacobs, PhD

When I was six weeks old, the so-named, "Korean war" broke out and my father, a US army physician at the time, was ordered to depart for Korea immediately. My mother then left the army base and moved into her mother's home, with me and my brother and in tow. My grandmother's circle of friends from the amateur theater company of which she was a part, included three men in particular, all gay, who were the men who held me, cuddled me and giggled with me for the first 18 months of my life. They remained special to me for many years.

No one ever mentioned the fact that these dear friends of my grandmother were gay. It had to be an open secret. They, and I, paid a price. We loved each other, but with a carefully calibrated intimacy.

Times have changed, as evidenced by this brave collection of writings. But times have *not* changed enough, as is also evidenced by this brave collection of writings! There are undertones in so many of these chapters, at some moments a plea to be accorded the same freedom to live their full humanity, a humanity that I, as a straight white woman am accorded to a greater degree (while not fully); and at other moments a defiance, an insistence that they will not be denied their freedom to live their full humanity. And there is a fierce determination to use their clinical and personal experience to help all of us develop a more welcoming and knowledgeable sex and gender affirmative consulting room for our patients.

There is no doubt that my patients will benefit from my having read this book. And I have benefitted personally. Some of the explorations have expanded my knowledge, some have challenged a few of my assumptions, especially explorations of sexuality. I have been invited to feel my way into a worldview that challenges the common binaries of gay/straight and male/female, among others. Once we open ourselves to a less binary view of any human experience, and we critique received norms about gender and sexuality, we are freer, fuller, more expansive, more fluid in how we welcome our patients, and also in how we understand ourselves. The experience of reading this book has changed me, and I am richer for it.

We all know by now that the ground from which our figures emerge is thoroughly culturally saturated. Our figures of interest carry the shadow of culturally defined norms and are shaped and limited by our lack of awareness of their normative nature. When we lose sight of how culture-bound our figure/ground process is, it is easy for those of us situated in "privileged" social positions to pathologize people who break the socially-sanctioned norms. We don't recognize the norms as norms, but rather, they are simply "how things are (supposed to be)". I have been given the gift of learning that my white American ground is not reality, but is, instead, a collection of norms. The gift has come from being allowed to read and converse with black authors, friends and colleagues who can see my ground more clearly than I, in part because they have been injured by white norms that are treated as "reality." And the same is true about this book. The authors have challenged me to be a better person, better clinician, and a freer person in my own body, by challenging how we define gender and sexuality, and that we strive to define it at all!

Welcome Everyone

Ayhan Alman, John Gillespie and Vikram Kolmannskog

We welcome those of you who are gestalt therapy students, fully trained gestalt therapists, trainers, or researchers as well as those of you who belong to other therapeutic traditions or none at all. We welcome those of you who are new to topics like this one, and those with a great deal of related experience. We welcome your bodies – bodies of all sizes, abilities, and challenges, whether visible or invisible. We welcome all ages. We welcome all faith traditions, including those who lost their faith or never had one. We welcome people of all ethnicities, including black people, brown people, indigenous people, people with mixed ethnicities and those who are not sure where they belong. We welcome people of all economic backgrounds and current situations. We welcome all the languages we bring and the many ways we speak and write English. We welcome people of all genders including people who identify as transgender, non-binary, genderqueer, and everyone for whom labels do not apply. We welcome all sexual and relationship orientations, including queer and straight, partnered, single, monogamous, polyamorous, or otherwise. We welcome each of you in all the rich complexity of your identity, including dimensions we have not mentioned. We honour each of you in this work we are undertaking, and we say WELCOME.[1]

The International Association for the Advancement of Gestalt Therapy (IAAGT) hosts a biannual conference for gestalt practitioners. In 2018 in Toronto, during a conference themed 'Radical Respect' and focused on diversity, many (not all) queer identified gestalt therapists experienced something collectively which is hard to put in words. Hodgson[2] movingly describes one of her personal experiences:

> At the end of the opening evening there was an acknowledgement of men supporting women to attend. The heteronormativity was striking. As a lesbian I felt marginalised and excluded. I remained silent. I looked around to see if anyone else had reacted: not obviously, so I felt my isolation even more. The moment highlighted a very difficult theme, that of how to speak up whilst being alert to the risk of shaming the other.

The tension between silence and speaking up, the burden of isolation versus the risk of shaming the other is a prevalent theme for marginalised communities. This is where the idea for this book emerged from: a rigid gestalt that hurts queer communities.

The idea for this book started, after the conference, within the Gender and Sexual Diversity (GSD) special interest group of the IAAGT and moved with John Gillespie's support into the New Gestalt Voices community. We, the editors, have invited people from within and beyond the gestalt therapy communities to contribute, most of whom themselves identify as queer.

We are aware that all three editors are male presenting. This is a limitation that we have tried to mitigate by consciously inviting a wide range of contributors, not least folks who don't identify as male. Still, we have ended up with a majority of male authors. It should also be mentioned that many more perspectives, experiences and reflections could have been included in an anthology on Gender, Sex and Relationship Diversity (GSRD).[3] At some point, we had to start working with the contributions that we had, however, and we do believe that this book is a substantial addition to the field - and hopefully, many more will come.

As indicated in our opening paragraph, this book is for everyone who is interested in GSRD and therapy, especially gestalt therapy. Everyone regardless of gender identity, sexual orientation or relationship preferences. While we warmly welcome readers who belong to other therapeutic traditions or none at all, you should know that several chapters do take for granted a basic understanding of gestalt therapy theory and concepts. There are a range of other books that can work as introductions to gestalt therapy and we refer the interested readers to these.[4] This book is also an invitation to further queer the gestalt community with diverse content ranging from academic, research-oriented pieces to experiential, reflective perspectives. While appreciating academic rigour, we know academia itself excludes many voices that are worthy of being heard. This is why we put all chapters through a peer review process but eventually prioritised experience over theory, vulnerability over perfection, accessibility over limitation.

While recognising that many chapters present and explore the complexity of GSRD, we have chosen to structure the book by starting with chapters that focus on gender (Morrison's Gender Radical Clients, Almås', Hosemans', Palmou's, Waletich's); followed by those focused on sex and sexuality (Grace's, Ricketts', Kumar's, Neves'); then one on relationship diversity (Morrison's Queering Relationships); ending with three overarching, general chapters: one on secret LGBTI lives in rural Ireland (Desmond's), one on integrating GSRD and gestalt therapy (Alman's), and another on addressing heteronormativity in gestalt therapy training (Kolmannskog's).

It has taken us four long years to complete this book project. It was a community effort with countless volunteers who put their hearts, minds, and bodies into this project to get it over the finish line. It has certainly influenced and enriched us, the editors, personally and professionally. Our hope is that you, the reader, will experience provocation, curiosity, familiarity, excitement and not least continue to learn and grow and help make gestalt therapy and other fields more GSRD-sensitive.

Notes

1 This welcome is inspired by 'Canticle – We Welcome You' which Vikram came across as a student in the Mindfulness Meditation Teacher Certification Programme (https://mmtcp.soundstrue.com/)
2 Hodgson, D. (2018). Reflections on radical respect. *British Gestalt Journal* 27/29, (62–63).
3 The term 'Gender & Sexual Diversity' was originally coined by Sexologist Dominic Davies (2007) and further developed to 'Gender, Sexuality & Relationship Diversity' (GSRD) by Dr MJ Barker (Davies & Barker, 2015). Davies graciously told us in an email the latest iteration of the term GSRD changed the word 'Sexuality' to 'Sex' for more inclusivity of intersex lived experiences because the term sex can mean 'sexuality' and 'biological sex' (see also Davies & Pink Therapy, 2021).
4 One of the editors, Vikram Kolmannskog, has written a book that is both a collection of therapy tales and an introduction to gestalt therapy: *The Empty Chair. Tales from Gestalt Therapy* (Routledge, 2018).

References

Davies, D., 2007. Not in Front of the Students. *Therapy Today: BACP*. 18.

Davies, D. and Barker, M. J., 2015. Gender and Sexual Diversity: respecting difference. *The Psychotherapist*. 60, 16–17.

Davies, D. and Pink Therapy, 2021. *What does GSRD mean?* [online] available at: https://pinktherapy.org/gsrd_en/ [accessed 25/05/2022].

Hodgson, D. (2018). Reflections on radical respect. *British Gestalt Journal* 27(29), 62–63.

Kolmannskog, V. (2018). *The Empty Chair. Tales from Gestalt Therapy*. Routledge.

Chapter 1

Understanding Gender Radical Clients

Daniel Morrison

The term gender radical is used here to mean anyone who isn't cisgender. Cisgender, or cis, refers to a person who identifies as the gender they were assigned at birth. When they were born, the doctor said, 'it's a girl' or 'it's a boy' and they've never felt uncomfortable with that. It can be difficult for some cis people to find they have a label, but it's just a descriptive word that exists so we can talk about people who are not gender radical without using words like 'normal', 'natural' or 'real'. Transgender and gender radical people are all of these things as well. Other terms often used for gender radical people include gender non-conforming, gender diverse, or trans*. The issue with these terms is that they have some degree of ambiguity or are not specific enough. A butch lesbian could be described as gender non-conforming in that she performs femininity in a way that is not traditional, but she may strongly identify as female. Gender diversity includes the whole spectrum of gender, including cisgender people. Trans* seems to centre binary trans people and is a word some nonbinary or genderfluid people feel doesn't apply to them and is therefore to some degree excluding. Gender radical or gender creative are non-pathologising and celebratory terms, but it should be noted that cisgender people can approach or express their gender in ways that are radical and creative as well. This is a field that is evolving, and the words we have are often not right for everyone. It's difficult to find a term that's specific enough to effectively describe the group of individuals we're talking about, without excluding some elements of that group. I've chosen to use gender radical here but also want to note that it's a term that people can choose to apply or not to apply to themselves.

Fundamental to the understanding of gender radical clients is the concept that when we use the terms gender or sex synonymously, we are conflating several distinct elements that may or may not be related. Biological sex refers to the physical body, gender expression to the way a person chooses to be and act in the world, and gender identity is an internal sense of self. None of these elements are binary, and although there is a correlation they are not inherently connected. Sexuality is separate and distinct from all these things and is beyond the scope of this chapter, beyond a brief acknowledgment that

DOI: 10.4324/9781003335344-1

a gender radical person can be lesbian, gay, asexual, bisexual, pansexual, heterosexual, queer or use another word to describe their orientation. The Gender Unicorn is a great visual aid to understanding this, presenting each of these axes as sliding scales independent of one another and representing biological sex as the body, gender expression as the outward appearance and gender identity in the mind, and can be found here: www.transstudent.org/gender.

Biological Sex

The first thing to understand is that biological sex is different from gender, although these words are often used interchangeably. The separation of the two can feel like mental yoga if it's the first time you've come across it but is the foundation of understanding gender radical clients.

Biological sex is based on many different things, hormones, external genitals, secondary sexual characteristics, genetics, brain structure and chemistry, and others. It's generally understood that each characteristic is like two buckets, two binary options, either this or that, which correlate with gender. For example, a person with XX chromosomes will have a vulva, grow breasts at puberty, produce oestrogen and progesterone and refer to herself as a woman. The trouble is that when you look at any one of these characteristics, there are exceptions. There are over a thousand different intersex conditions, many of which people never know they have. Intersex is not a gender identity, it refers to a nonbinary biological sex.

One way to look at this is using height. It's an obvious and provable fact that men are taller than women, but if a tall woman stands next to a short man, she's taller than he is. On seeing that, we don't say that it's not true that men are taller than women. We don't say, they must be wrong about their gender or we must be reading their gender wrong. The conclusion we draw would be that generally men are taller than women, but some women are taller than some men. There are exceptions, and we're comfortable with having a rule that doesn't apply in all cases.

The same applies for other aspects of biological sex. Generally, men have penises but not always. A cis man may have lost his penis due to accident, injury or illness. A trans man may have been born without one. An intersex man may have genitals that are ambiguous but identify himself as male. A trans woman may have or once have had a penis but is not a man. In the same way, it's true that most people with breasts are women but not always. The examples above apply equally; a woman who has lost her breasts to illness is of course still a woman, but a difference here is that the distinction is more obviously socially conditioned and informed by the sexualisation of women's bodies. A cis man with a larger build often has more breast tissue than a slim cis woman, but his gender is not questioned and neither is his right to be topless in public.

Cisgender people modify their bodies in many of the same ways that gender radical people do. Hormones are routinely prescribed for contraception, menopause, sexual dysfunction, acne, PMT and other reasons. Cis women may have breast reduction or enhancement surgery. Gynecomastia is a condition where cis men develop excessive breast tissue, which is treated with hormones or surgery, in exactly the same way as it is for trans men.

Physics shows us that even solid objects are, at the atomic level, made mostly of empty space. We can hold that knowledge while still interacting with the world around us as if it were real and solid. Even a quantum physicist will put her coffee down on a table, not on thin air. In the same way, the words 'man' and 'woman', 'male' and 'female' are useful shorthand that work for most people most of the time. Gender and biological sex are two separate concepts that usually correlate but sometimes don't. Like consensus reality, the more closely gender and biological sex are examined, the more exceptions we find until there are so many empty spaces we question whether it exists at all.

At the time of writing, 2,617 scientists had signed an open letter saying that "the relationship between sex chromosomes, genitalia, and gender identity is complex, and not fully understood. There are no genetic tests that can unambiguously determine gender, or even sex." Signatories include biologists, geneticists, psychologists, anthropologists, physicians, neuroscientists, social scientists, biochemists, mental health service providers and nine Nobel prize winners. The full letter can be read here: www.not-binary.org/statement/.

Gender Identity

Gender identity is an internal sense of self and is not something that can be seen from the outside. Everyone has a gender identity, not just gender radical people. Sometimes gender identity is binary, male or female, which may or may not match the gender assigned at birth. Sometimes it's more complex, fluid or non-existent.

The way gender identity is usually communicated is by pronouns. Pronouns are the words we use instead of repeating a name, for example "Kim has gone to get her pen". We all use pronouns and those who feel comfortable with the pronouns used for them have usually never given much thought to it. Pronouns are he, she or they, which is grammatically correct for one person. 'They' has been used as a singular gender neutral pronoun by Shakespeare, Chaucer and Austen, and is in general use today in situations where a person doesn't know the gender of the person they're talking about. Did you notice its use in that sentence, or elsewhere in this chapter? Other pronouns are sometimes used, such as que, ze or hir. Pronouns broadly correlate to gender identity – someone who uses he pronouns will usually be comfortable being thought of as male, those who use she pronouns are generally comfortable with a female identity, but those who use other pronouns are not inviting more discussion or assumptions about their gender identity. Using other pronouns may mean simply that their gender is 'other' and they may not want to explain the subtleties and nuances of their experience. When meeting a new person, we don't assume their name and think they're being awkward or difficult if they tell us it's something else. If we've recently met a group of people, we might make an internal effort to remember their names, perhaps repeating names in our heads or asking again those we can't remember. If asking pronouns rather than assuming them was normalised in the same way, and if everyone accepted that remembering pronouns was their work to do, the world would be a much more welcoming place for gender radical people. There are some other practical ideas in the box below of ways to work with conditioning and open up conversations about why this is important.

Pronoun Problems: How to Change Your Mind

- Try making a running commentary in your head while with the person, or watching a video clip of someone who uses unfamiliar pronouns – "Ze is getting a mug. Ze is putting the kettle on. Ze is talking about hir job."
- Notice when you or others use they as a singular pronoun when you don't know the gender of the person.
- Notice assumptions about gender – when a car overtakes you, do you think 'he's going too fast'? Could you change that to 'they are going too fast'?
- Consider using your pronouns on your email signature.
- Introduce yourself using your pronouns when holding a group and invite others to do so.
- Think about pets – when meeting someone's dog, it's easy to ask 'he or she?' and accept it if your assumption is corrected.

Gender identity is complex and difficult to define, being an internal and internalised sense of self that is unique to each individual. There is valuable personal work to be done for everyone in exploring this. Is a cisgender identity of 'male' or 'female' conditioned and habitual, or an authentic expression of self? What does such an identity open up, and what does it close down? How has it affected the individual's life, and how would it be different if gendered conditioning was not present in their culture? This richness of discovery is something most gender radical people have access to, which can be of great benefit in understanding their internal world. There are many excellent collections of writing by gender radical people willing to share this deeply personal experience, such as those edited by Morty Diamond (2005) and Declan Henry (2017). Therapists who want to work with gender radical clients should be encouraged to examine their own assumptions around gender to avoid unconscious prejudice becoming an issue in the therapy room. *How to Understand Your Gender* by Alex Iantaffi and Meg-John Barker (2017) and *Gender Outlaw* by Kate Bornstein (2016) are excellent starting points.

Gender Expression

Gender expression is a person's outward appearance and can vary from day to day. Gender may be expressed through clothes, hairstyle, body language or speech. It is separate from both biological sex and gender identity. A butch lesbian and a trans man may have the same gender expression, meaning the same style of clothes and hair, and the same biological sex assigned at birth, but their gender identity is different – one is a woman and the other is a man. This is the difference between a cross-dresser and a trans woman – a cross-dresser is a man who wears women's clothes some or all of the time; a trans woman is a woman who was assigned male at birth. Both are valid, and the difference between the two is in their internal sense of themselves. As with biological sex and gender identity, gender expression is not binary. Many people who identify themselves outside the gender binary present in a way that is androgynous but may also feel comfortable presenting in a more binary way, which may or may not correlate with their biological sex. A person who was assigned female at birth and presents in a traditionally 'female' way can have an internal sense of themselves as nonbinary, male, fluid or anything else. This may be through choice; they may feel comfortable with this presentation. It may be for convenience; they're not entirely comfortable but it's possible for them to present as female and makes their life easier. It may also be that they are forced to present in this way for their own safety, and this can cause a great deal of distress and incongruence.

The concept of 'passing' refers to the ability of a trans person to pass as cis and is problematic for many reasons. Trans women are policed based on their appearance and ability to 'pass' as cisgender women far more than trans men are, a discrepancy that has its roots in misogyny and the judgement of all women based on their appearance. Trans men benefit from the assumption that male is the default position unless there is evidence otherwise, as described below. A trans man with a beard is likely to 'pass' as cis-male, albeit an unusual looking one, even if he has other obvious signifiers that he was assigned female at birth. The term 'passing' suggests subterfuge and has failure as its antithesis. A different way to express the same idea is by describing how a person is 'read', how they are perceived by those around them. This puts the onus on to the observer and allows for the gender identity to be valid even if it doesn't match the outward appearance.

Labels and Identities

There are many words for different gender identities, and more are emerging all the time. When people begin to explore their sense of gender as separate from their biological sex, sometimes they find that there isn't a word to describe their experience so they find one, or make one up. Some of these words are new, but the experiences are not new. Gender radical people exist and have existed in all cultures and periods of history, and are often highly valued as leaders, spiritual guides, healers or magic workers. Leslie Feinberg's (1997) book *Transgender Warriors* explores the rich and hidden history of gender radical people across cultures. A binary essentialist view of gender is a modern invention. For a person who has always felt that there is something unidentifiable 'wrong' with them, finding a word that describes their experience can be hugely empowering and validating. There's a sense of 'I'm not broken, I'm not alone, there are other people like me.' Equally, some gender radical people choose not to use words to define themselves or their gender, finding labels restrictive or over complicated, or may feel internal or external pressure to choose a label.

You're invited to pause here for a moment, and imagine a person going down the street, not someone you know, just a person, a stranger. Make that mental image clear in your mind.

It's likely that the image is of a white man, walking. That tends to be the default position when we think of 'person'. To create a mental image of a woman, the word 'woman' would probably have to be used, and the mental image would probably be of a white woman unless something else was specified. To create a mental image of a Black trans woman in a wheelchair, we need more words. This is a useful illustration of why these labels are necessary. It's often said that we're all just people, there's no need to use all these labels, and the people who say that tend to be those who are closer to that default position of gender, race, ability and orientation.

Some labels that gender radical people use are described below, but it's important to note that the explanations are not definitions. These words may be chosen by people with different experiences and should be treated as a starting point for discussion in therapy, if the client chooses to do so. Identity politics is rife online and often vitriolic and damaging, and nobody has the right to police another's gender or the words they use to describe it. Phrases like 'not trans enough' or 'not looking nonbinary' can be deeply harmful and invalidating. Having said that, a general understanding of what terms might be used and what they might mean is essential in working with gender radical clients.

- "I don't really know what people mean by an internal sense of gender. I was assigned male at birth and don't mind he pronouns but I'm agender, or genderless"
- "I'm genderqueer, I dress in a way which makes people question their assumptions about gender and don't feel male or female. My pronouns are ze/hir."
- "I'm a nonbinary trans man and use he/him pronouns. For me that means that I want to medically transition and be read as male, but inside I don't feel male or female."
- "I'm genderfluid. Some days I feel like a boy and some days like girl, and I dress according to how I feel on the day. My pronouns are they."
- "I am a woman with a trans history. I use she pronouns and have had all the medical intervention I want and consider my transition complete."
- "I'm nonbinary, I use they pronouns and wear androgynous clothes. I feel about 60% male and 40% female."

Gender Dysphoria

Gender dysphoria is a specific term for a particular kind of incongruence relating to gender. It can be physical, relating to gendered parts of the body, or it can be social, relating to the way people are treated in the world depending on whether they are perceived as male or female, or both. Not all gender radical people experience dysphoria, and not all who do, experience it in the same way. Gender dysphoria could be a subtle sense of not being quite comfortable, of something being slightly wrong all the time, or it could be crippling, causing the person so much distress they can't leave the house. It can and often does lead to suicide, self-harm or self-medicating using drugs or alcohol. It's not a mental health condition. The treatment is medical transition and as this happens, generally dysphoria is brought to a manageable level or cured completely if the person has a binary gender identity. The role of the therapist is in some ways the same as for any other presentation of incongruence, supporting the client and holding space. The difference of course is that for gender radical people who want to transition there will be a medical process that allows this to happen as well as the psychological process.

For gender radical people with a binary gender identity, that is, who identify as male or female, or are comfortable being perceived as one of these, medical transition is likely to help with their dysphoria. Those with nonbinary gender identities, including agender, genderqueer, genderfluid and others, may find that there isn't a way for them to be perceived as they are in their everyday life. Cultural conditioning means that a binary view of gender is the norm and anything outside that brings discomfort and is assigned to one or other binary gender. It may be that some level of medical intervention such as low dose hormones enables the person to inhabit the space between binary genders and be read as sometimes male and sometimes female. This may be comfortable for some gender radical people but is difficult to maintain in the long term, as the effect of hormones is cumulative so they will tend to appear 'more male' or 'more female' over time. The choice to pursue some aspects of medical transition without others presents additional barriers when navigating a system that is still based largely on an assumption of binary gender identities.

It is possible that the hardest part of transitioning, and the part where people are at the highest risk of suicide, are the years when they are waiting for medical treatment. In the UK, General Practitioners (GPs) refer patients to a Gender Identity Clinic, and the waiting list may be years before the first appointment. Some GPs are reluctant to refer where there are existing mental health conditions, they aren't aware of the process of referral or of the appropriate way to treat gender radical clients. Race, disability, education and social situation can also create additional barriers when navigating the healthcare system. Gender radical people must present as their gender for one to two years before being able to access professional support from a Gender Identity Clinic, which is uncomfortable at best and dangerous at worst. Generally two appointments with psychiatrists are necessary, which may be several months apart, before a diagnosis of gender dysphoria is made and hormones can be prescribed. Surgery may require an additional wait of several years. The effect of this is that even binary gender radical people face a period of several years when they are typically read as their biological sex assigned at birth but are forced to be 'out' in all situations as their real gender whether they choose to or not. For a more detailed explanation of the process of medical transition, Ben Vincent's (2018) book *Transgender Health* is recommended.

Intersectionality and Transphobia

The fact that gender radical people face repeated psychiatric assessment and years of waiting lists to access medical treatment that is easily accessible to cisgender people highlights the inequalities that are inherent in the system. This incongruence arises from transphobia. When all the other reasons for denying healthcare and recognition are examined and removed, as we are doing here, any remaining objection must be seen as irrational and arising from fear and prejudice. Gender radical people are regularly demonised and misrepresented by the media, and misconceptions abound even in some people who consider themselves allies.

Genital surgery is commonly performed on babies whose gender is ambiguous at birth, often without the knowledge or consent of the parents. There is public outrage about trans young people and teenagers being too young to understand or consent to the permanent changes from long-term hormone use but none about this routine practice. The intersex community campaign to raise awareness and opposition to permanent and non-consensual genital surgery on new-born babies is met with indifference, but a young person whose parents agree to them taking hormones receives national coverage.

Barriers to accessing support and medical care arise from racial prejudice, as Black or Asian trans men are perceived as dangerous when they begin to be read as male. Fatal violence disproportionately affects trans women of colour, in addition to prejudice affecting other risk factors such as access to housing, jobs and education.

Disabled people regularly have to choose between accessing healthcare as a disabled person or as a gender radical person, or risk having their health-care needs marginalised by their gender identity. 'Trans broken arm syndrome' refers to mainstream medical professionals refusing to treat routine healthcare issues because they don't specialise in gender issues.

Gender Radical Clients in Therapy

Gender radical clients may be broadly grouped into three types, in terms of presenting issues and the goals of therapy. The first of these, and perhaps the most likely to be encountered by non-specialists, are those clients who don't yet know that they are experiencing gender dysphoria. These clients may arrive in the therapy room with a general sense of incongruence, distress, something not being right, which they may have self-medicated with alcohol or drugs, or might express as anxiety or depression, or perfectionism, work addiction or unhealthy relationship patterns – in essence, anything that any other client, or person, might come across in their lives. In this case it's essential that therapists are aware of gender as a possibility and notice the first tentative suggestions that clients may offer. Many gender radical people have a therapy horror story of a thoughtless comment by a therapist when they were opening up their box of gender issues, which closed them down and ended therapy, often for years.

A second group of clients are those who are aware that their gender is an issue they want to explore with the support of a therapist. It's likely that such a client would seek out a therapist who lists gender diversity as a particular area of experience.

A third group may be clients who are comfortable and secure in their gender identity, having done their therapeutic work and possibly their medical transition. A trans history indicates that a person considers their medical transition complete. A binary trans woman who has had all the medical interventions she wants may refer to herself as a woman with a trans history when she wants to distinguish herself from cisgender women. The client with a trans history who is experiencing relationship difficulties, or the nonbinary person who is comfortable inhabiting the liminal space between and outside gender but is experiencing unrelated mental health issues, might fall into this third group. No specialist knowledge of working with gender radical clients is necessary in this case, as it's not the presenting issue nor the underlying cause. It's important here that the therapist doesn't make the assumption that the underlying cause for other unrelated issues is that the client is gender radical in some way.

The principles of gestalt therapy are conducive to effective work with gender radical clients, as the underlying concept is that of meeting clients where they are and working on their current situation. The difference when working with gender radical clients is that therapists may have unexamined assumptions operating around gender that interfere with their ability to do this. Certain elements of gestalt therapy might be particularly useful, such as empty chair work with clients who feel they have a 'male self' and a 'female self'. Hearing both these voices, and enabling them to communicate with one another, could be a rich source of therapeutic exploration. Similarly, inner child work where the child is a different gender to the adult could be invaluable. A transmasculine person's inner child could be male although the person as a child was read as female, or could be experienced as female and representing the previous female self. Some people who have transitioned genders or are in the process of doing so experience loss or grief for their 'old self' who may be disappearing. Some may have deep injuries from years or decades of hiding who they really are, or of being misgendered throughout their lives. Narratives of being 'trans enough' may be threatened by the presence of inner voices with different gender identities, or internalised misogyny, misandry or transphobia may cause some aspects of the gendered self to be rejected or silenced. Therapeutic work that enables the client to express their various selves may bring resolution to such structures, allowing a gestalt to be completed.

Conclusion

The point here is that the experience of everyday reality is at odds with the facts. A cisgender person's social world and culture is likely to be largely populated by other cisgender people – their friends and family, the people they interact with and the images they see online and on TV will be almost entirely cisgender, or apparently so. Their lived experience is that biological sex equates to gender, and there may be nothing in their life that contradicts this assumption. This is comfortable and familiar and therefore seems natural and true. It takes mental effort and a willingness to be uncomfortable to go beyond this, and there is often resistance and fear to the challenge brought by opening up our understanding. As therapists, it's essential that we are willing to meet this challenge and explore what it brings up in us. If a physicist explained that solid objects in the world were in fact mostly empty space at the atomic level and was met by ridicule and disbelief by an individual, it would probably not concern them too much. They would be able to shrug and move on with their life. The difference with gender radical people is that the incongruity of their biological sex with their gender is their lived experience, and to fail to hear their voice is to deny their very existence and validity as human beings.

About Daniel Morrison

Daniel Morrison is a psychotherapist in the UK. He specialises in working with clients around gender diversity, ethical nonmonogamy and neurodiversity. He also facilitates workshops on connection and polyvagal theory, supporting participants to learn about their autonomic nervous system and offering practical tools to manage and improve mental health. He is a writer, parent, Queer activist and performer. As a neuroqueer nonbinary trans man he brings his own lived experience to his client work, offering relational and integrative trauma informed therapy.

References

Bornstein, K. (2016). *Gender Outlaw: On Men, Women and the Rest of Us*. Vintage.

Diamond, M. (2005). *From the Inside Out: Radical Gender Transformation, FTM and Beyond*. Manic D Press, U.S.

Feinberg, L. (1997). *Transgender Warriors*, Beacon Press.

Henry, D. (2017). *Trans Voices: Becoming Who You Are*. Jessica Kingsley Publishers.

Iantaffi, A. and Barker, M.-J. (2017). *How to Understand Your Gender: A Practical Guide for Exploring Who You Are*. Jessica Kingsley Publishers.

Vincent, B. (2018). *Transgender Health: A Practitioner's Guide to Binary and Non-Binary Trans Patient Care*. Jessica Kingsley Publishers.

Chapter 2

Gender Identification

Elsa Almås

A "Modern" Trans

Around 2007 I met the first person that I came to call a "modern" trans in my therapy room (Plummer, 1991). Perhaps "modern" gives confusing signals in a post post-modern time but let us just look at the original meaning of modern, which includes new, being able to shape oneself, free, based on knowledge, re-examining every aspect of existence (for a short introduction, see Wikipedia). The first "modern" trans in my office was soon followed by several, characterized first of all by lack of shame; they were self-confident, had support from friends and family, were educated, or still in school or university, some were in jobs – most of them were young. Some had been in psychiatric treatment but found it absurd; one was even working as psychologist himself.

I was better prepared than many therapists to meet these "modern" trans people, as I had been married to EE, a trans person, since 1988. I have been fortunate to live close to, and even inside the trans community since 1986, and I have seen the development of the professional community, the trans community and the society at large; how the phenomenon we call "trans" has grown out of the binary model into variations of nature along several proposed dimensions of gender: neurophysiological, psychologic, social, cultural, sexual.

Our brains can be more or less flexible and can render us more or less fit to adapt to societal norms. Individuals perceive their gender identity as an inner experience, something not chosen, but just has to be: I *am* male, female, trans, not gendered, non-binary. This knowledge cannot be detected from the outside, by identifying chromosomes, genitalia, hormones. It is a part of consciousness, like intelligence and musicality.

Variation in gender- and sexual identity are first of all represented by the diversity of self-experiences among individuals who regard themselves as gender variant.

DOI: 10.4324/9781003335344-2

When Facebook asked their users to define their gender by their own words, it resulted in 58 different definitions (Bivens, 2017). An American study among the transgender population published in 2016 asked the respondents to define their gender identity. This resulted in 500 new gender terms. Between 27 and 31 per cent identified as non-binary, gender queer or gender variant. In total, 20 per cent defined themselves as gender fluid, 18 per cent as androgyne (James et al., 2016). A Canadian study shows that 41 per cent of younger trans people regarded themselves as non-binary (Clark et al., 2019).

Different Understandings of Sex and Gender in History

Several paradigmatic changes have affected the understanding of sex, gender, and sex/gender identity. Some, like Michel Foucault, would say that sex and gender are products of society (Foucault, 1976/1980). Suraya Monro discusses postmodern/poststructuralist theories, arguing for a pluralist model of gender that supports intersex, androgynous, gender-fluid, transsexual, cross-dressing, multiply-gendered, and non-male/female people as:

1 physical, embodied people, with the biological foundationalism that this implies;
2 social people, who may change genders despite having fairly static physical appearance;
3 psychological people, who may have an experience of themselves which is different from their social and physical identities and mainstream male/female norms;
4 political actors, who require changes in social structures and institutions to enable them to have basic human rights;
5 academics, who may seek to critique current gender theory and develop pluralist alternatives.

(Monro, 2005, p. 14)

There are many possible controversies on a path leading towards a new theory of gender; concepts like "identity", "self", "gender as performance", and "biological foundationalism" are discussed – all controversies are possible sources of new insight. In the effort to develop a theory of gender that includes all variations, we must strive for a wider horizon, not a narrower one.

Three Genders

One of the earlier descriptions of gender is by Plato (429–347 BC), in *The Symposium*, presenting a group of the most distinguished intellectuals of Athens about 400 years BC, giving their respective speeches in praise of love. In his speech, Aristophanes, a famous actor in Athens, is telling the story about the androgynes, who lived "long time ago", in a time where human beings were not two genders, but three. The androgynes had four legs and four arms and two faces:

> The reason why there were these three genders, and why they were as described, is that the parents of the male gender were originally the sun, that of the female gender the earth, that of the combined gender the moon, because the moon is a combination of the sun and earth.
>
> (p. 27) (Plato, 1987/1999/2009)

A third gender is also present in ancient Asian culture, exemplified by a Shiva gestalt Ardhanarishvara with a body that is half male and half female. In more than hundred cultures studied by anthropologists, the combination of both male and female talents were regarded as necessary qualifications to receive training to become shaman (Dragoin, 1995).

The One Sex and Two Sex Models

Changes in social and political circumstances have for centuries given men a privileged position. This was supported by the one-sex model, where women were regarded as less developed than men. The development of the two-sex model is described by Thomas Laqueur in his book *Making Sex* (Laqueur, 1990/2001). In the introduction Laqueur describes how sexuality was affected by the development of the two-sex model:

> I discovered early on that the erasure of female pleasure from medical accounts of conception took place roughly at the same time as the female body came to be understood no longer as a lesser version of the male's (a one-sex model) but as its incommensurable opposite (a two-sex model) (Preface viii).
>
> (Laqueur, 1990/2001)

Medicalization of Sex and Gender

The first modern descriptions of gender expressions outside the binary model, using the word "trans", were introduced by medical doctors a little more than hundred years ago (Hirschfeld, 1910/1991; von Krafft-Ebing, 1886/1997), followed by the influence of psychoanalytic understanding of sex and gender (Freud, 1905/2000). Along with the interest of the psychoanalysts, came an understanding that gender identity that is not congruent with the sex assigned at birth, was the result of developmental influences, particularly identification with the parents as models of being male or female, and labelled as a *sexual deviance* (De Block & Adriaens, 2013). In the book *Die Transvestiten* published in 1910, Hirschfeld described the sex differences in four categories:

1 The sexual organs.
2 The other physical characteristics.
3 The sex drive.
4 The other emotional characteristics.

A complete womanly and "absolute" woman would be such a one who not only produces egg cells but also corresponds to the womanly type in every other aspect; an absolute man would be such a one who forms semen cells yet also, at the same time, exhibits the manly average type in all other point.

(Hirschfeld, 1910, p. 219)

Hirschfeld continues by describing how individuals correspond to these criteria to different degrees. He develops a mathematical model to account for possible combinations, ending up with 43 046 721 (Hirschfeld, 2010, p. 227).

Gender Diversity

At the beginning of the twentieth century, European culture was reflecting extreme differences between men and women. The polarization of the roles of men and women in society were based on the centrality of reproduction and protection of men's exclusive right to own property on behalf of the family.

The struggle for women's rights has been an important forerunner to the struggle for broader gender equality! The feminist movement had already challenged the traditional understanding of femininity and masculinity as innate. In 1949, the French writer and philosopher Simone de Beauvoir published *The Second Sex*, challenging the traditional view of sex (the concept of gender had not yet been introduced); her main statement was that *we are not born women, we become women*! This statement says that femaleness is something we learn. She also challenged the idea of reproduction as strictly binary, showing that procreation in nature takes many forms, and that it does not necessarily involve a male and a female zygote. Simone de Beauvoir questioned the idea that to be a woman is to procreate, and that her purpose in life is to serve the man in the continuation of his ancestry.

Introduction of the Word "Gender"

According to Milton Diamond, "the first known use of the word gender was listed as 1387 CE when T. Usk wrote 'No mo genders been there but masculine and femynyne, all the remnaunte been no genders but of grace, in faculte of grammar' *(Simpson & Weiner, 1989)*" (Diamond, 2002), but it is John Money who has been credited with having introduced the concept *gender* into the English vocabulary as the psychological and social expression of being a boy/man, or girl/woman (Money, 1952). Based on research on a group of intersex individuals he defined gender role as "all those things a person says or does to disclose himself or herself as having the status of boy or man, girl or woman, respectively. It includes but is not restricted to sexuality in the sense of eroticism" () (Money et al., 1955, p. 302). They concluded that gender role could not be attributed to chromosomal sex, gonadal sex, hormonal sex or genital morphology. They found a close consistency between assigned sex and rearing, and gender role and orientation as boy or girl, man or woman. Their conclusion was that "sexual behavior and orientation as male or female does not have an instinctive basis" (Money et al., 1955, p. 308), but "This statement is not an endorsement of a simple-minded theory of social and environmental determinism. Experiences are transacted, as well as encountered – conjunction of the two terms is imperative – and encounters do not automatically dictate predictable transactions" (Money et al., 1955, p. 310).

The common idea in sexology became that gender identity was based on the assigned gender at birth and the parent's upbringing in accordance with this assignment. This is why John Money found it important to surgically correct genitals that did not seem to be strictly male or female, in order to secure what was regarded as a healthy binary gender identity.

Milton Diamond questioned the validity of basing a general theory about gender identity on findings from intersex individuals. Diamond did not go back to instinct theories but claimed that there must be an innate element as a basis for the subjective experience of gender identity. He based much of his arguments on brain research, but never actually presented an explanatory model for the subjective experience of gender identity.

The Introduction of Trans

Harry Benjamin writes:

> For the simple man in the street, there are only two sexes. A person is either male or female, Adam or Eve. With more learning comes more doubt [...] With the advancement of biologic and especially genetic studies, the concept of "male" and "female" has become rather uncertain. There is no longer an absolute division (dichotomy). The dominant status of the genital organs for the determination of one's sex has been shaken, at least in the world of science.
>
> (Benjamin, 1966, pp. 6–7)

The differentiation between *transsexuals*, who refused to live as the assigned gender, and *transvestites*, who were usually men who occasionally liked to dress up as women, was defined by the extent of departure from the assigned sex at birth. Both groups were offered psychotherapy, without success. After years of attempts to treat what was regarded as a delusion, Harry Benjamin challenged the psycho-pathologizing of transsexuality: "Since it is evident, therefore, that the mind of the transsexual cannot be adjusted to the body, it is logical and justifiable to attempt the opposite. To adjust the body to the mind" (Benjamin, 1966, p. 53).

In 1995, EE and I attended the first *International Congress on Gender, Cross Dressing and Sex Issues* in Van Nuys, California. A second congress was held in King of Prussia in Philadelphia in 1997, and a third congress on sex and gender in Oxford in 1998. At these congresses gender variant individuals were present as professionals discussing gender diversity based on a non-pathological approach. We met philosophers, anthropologists, linguists, artists, as well as psychologists, urologists, psychiatrists who were dismissing pathologizing diagnoses, shame and isolation, defining themselves as what they were with pride.

I was attending the conferences as a psychologist and a sexologist, but most of all I was included and given credentials by being wife of a trans person. I was impressed by the number of outstanding artists and performers gathered at a private garden party after one of the conferences: There were composers, musicians and conductors as well as shamans, medical doctors, psychologists, researchers and writers in different academic and non-academic fields. That was where I first started to replace the word *co-morbidity* with *co-capacity*, and EE introduced the word *trans talent*! Being trans was in this setting far from a disturbance or something dysphoric – it was indeed a talent accompanied by many co-talents, pride and ambitions to use these talents to explore and understand trans-phenomena better!

In 1997, basic ideas for understanding trans people were hit by a major blow that challenged the general understanding of sex and gender. We had witnessed a conflict between the two giants for many years: John Money and Milton Diamond. The conflict was based on disagreement about how gender identity is established and developed. John Money's theory, about genitals and rearing (Money & Ehrhardt, 1972; Money et al., 1955), was challenged by the publication of what really happened in the famous John/Joan case.

In the John/Joan case a boy child who lost his penis during circumcision had been medically transformed into a "girl". The "girl" had, however, never adapted to a female gender role but had been depressed, unhappy, and over-weight when "she" received female hormones to initiate puberty. She insisted on peeing standing and playing with boys' toys (Diamond & Sigmundson, 1997). We met Milton Diamond and Keith Sigmundsson in Hawaii in 1998, and Sigmundsson, who had been supervising the therapists working with Joan, as the child was named, explained that one day a young female psychiatrist in training came out from the therapy room, saying, *"But this is not a girl, it is a boy!"* Sigmundsson said that this was like when the little boy in H.C. Andersons fairy tale said, *"But the Emperor has no clothes!"* They decided to tell the little "girl", now 14 years of age, about her background, and "she" decided that "she" wanted to go back to being the boy she had been born as – and felt like! The history of John/Joan was published in a paediatric journal in February 1997, causing an immediate article in *Time* magazine in March 1997 and in the music magazine *Rolling Stone* (December, 1997) by John Colapinto, who later also published a book about the story (Colapinto, 2000).

For me, the publication of the John/Joan story was a relief, as it made much more sense that gender identity is more basic than what can be constructed by rearing and culture. Trans persons themselves describe the feeling of having a gender identity that does not fit their bodies as a very strong sensation that comes from within. In the wake of the publication, a consensus-report about "Atypical Gender Development" was published in 2006 summarizing the consensus in 45 points. In point 28 in this report, the experts wrote about the John/Joan case.

This case was, for many years, believed to support the view that, in instances of ambiguity of genitalia at birth or their accidental damage shortly thereafter, a child's gender identity could be largely determined by rearing, so long as this was consistent with the external sex characteristics. Infants were regarded as psychosexually neutral up to the age of two (Money and Ehrhardt, 1972), so reassignment had to be achieved before that age. However, later follow-up revealed that the attempt to impose a female gender identity on John failed. Despite psychological treatment to make him more comfortable in the female role, Joan reverted to being John during adolescence; he married and became stepfather to his wife's children (Diamond & Sigmundson, 1997; Besser et al., 2006; Kipnis & Diamond, 1998; Colapinto, 2000).

Understanding sex and gender in our culture is based on the idea of sexual dimorphism, but as Harry Benjamin indicated, this dimorphism is far from absolute. One person can be equipped with genitals consisting of both male and female characteristics, which has been named hermaphrodite, and intersex; have mosaics of chromosomes, or half of the cells in the body can have XX chromosomes, and the other half can have XY chromosomes.

What is interpreted by the individual and by society as gender identity, does not necessary align with the genital appearance, and cannot necessarily be overridden by consistent socialization (Besser et al., 2006).

Gender Belonging

A way to understand sex and gender is to regard them as continua between binary and out of the binary expressions. In 1993, we published a paper in *Nordic Sexology* (*Nordisk Sexologi*) with the English title "Affirmation model for gender belonging" (Benestad & Almås, 1993). The basic idea is that positive gender belonging depends on affirmation from bodily, psychological as well as cultural mirroring. "Positive belonging arises as one is perceived as gender by others in the same way as one perceives oneself, and when that which is perceived is given a positive value" (Benestad, 2016, p. 97).

The differentiation is described on six levels, based on the observation that individuals can represent expressions of sex and gender on a fleeting scale between male and female:

1   *Somatic sex* equals external natal sex. This is not the same as *biological sex*, since the somatic body can contain biological markers that cannot be detected from the outside of the body.
2   *Gender identity* is the subjective experience of being gendered. The differentiations are: Male, female, trans/intersex or neither (those who dismiss gender).
3   *Body consciousness* is differentiated as experience of having a male, female, intersex or non-gendered body.
4   *Body picture* is divided into two sub-levels. One is *somatic body picture* with the differentiations male, female, intersex/hermaphrodite, or no sex characteristics. The other is *cultural body picture*, where the differentiations are feminine, masculine, androgyne, and not gendered.
5   *Gender role* is differentiated as male, female, androgyne, or neutral.
6   Erotic preference, differentiated into androphilic, gynephilic, androgynephilic, or not gendered preference.

(Benestad & Almås, 1993)

In 2015, Sari van Anders introduced the concept gender/sex as a self-experience that involves both biological and social dimensions; identity is linked to sexualities in what she denotes as a *sexual configuration*. She regards sexuality as part of a social context; sexuality is complex, and configurations can change. Van Anders introduces new definitions of old concepts: *Sexual attraction* involves sex/gender, age, status, norms, number of partners, type of sexual activity, intensity, single sex and consent. *Sexual orientation* involves sexual wishes and sexual needs, social role, affirmation, assurance, safety, being comfortable.

Sexual identities involve gender/sex sexualities (sexualities among individuals who experience gender incongruence, homo-curiosity, gender independent sexuality, un-gendered sex), normative, lesbian, gay, BDSM, fetish, polyamorous, asexual, player, mono-amorous, kink (van Anders, 2015).

In Anne Fausto-Sterling's 2019 publication, gender/sex, sexual orientation and identity are seen as elements in a larger system. Fausto-Sterling introduces the *orthogonal turn*, leaving behind the social-*versus*-nonsocial, nature-*versus*-nurture oppositions, outlining an approach that intertwines sex, gender, orientation, bodies, and cultures, without a demand to choose one over the other (Fausto-Sterling, 2019).

Our model of gender belonging is in accordance with the configuration model by van Anders, and the orthogonal turn described by Fausto-Sterling, and allows, as an example, for an individual to have a body that can be classified as a *male*, based on appearance, without knowledge about the biological internal configuration. This individual can have a *female gender identity*, experiencing a *male body consciousness*, presenting a male, with an andro-gyne body picture, having a *feminine gender role*, and be *attracted to women*.

Challenges for the Future

Trans activist are by their mere existence challenging traditional understand-ings of sex and gender. The binary sex/gender model as well as bio-medical understanding of normality and deviation, health and disease are challenged. New knowledge about epi-genetic processes suggests interaction between genes and environmental influences as a possible explanation of how gen-der identity can develop (Champagne, 2010). S. J. Langer suggests an inter-action between genome and environment, as a constellation of factors that may constitute gender identity (Langer, 2019). This theory is supported by network medicine (Silbersweig & Loscalzo, 2017). Rametti and Rametti, and Zhou et al. have described brain differences that indicate similarities in brains between cis- and trans females, and cis- and trans-males (Rametti et al., 2011; Zhou et al., 1995).

Trans individuals have, in line with research, showed that:

1   Gender identity is based on subjective experience;
2   Trans individuals do not necessarily hate their genitals, many use them for sexual pleasure;
3   Trans individuals are demonstrating gender euphoria and pride in being themselves as a variation of human diversity; and
4   Experience of gender incongruence is resolved in different ways for dif-ferent individuals, for some it is resolved by hormonal and surgical body modification (to different degrees), for others it is resolved by acceptance by society and acknowledgment of gender diversity.

ICD-11

An important and positive development is the de-psychiatrization of trans by the International Classification of Diseases (ICD-11), developed by the World Health Organization (WHO), and the introduction of the concept *gender incongruence* as an attempt to develop less stigmatizing medical lan-guage than *gender dysphoria*, or *gender identity disorder*.

The revision of ICD-11 has been paralleled by development of self-affir-mation in the trans communities, and by trans individuals entering the pro-fessional scene and introducing trans subjective perspectives.

Sex and Gender as Complex Phenomena

The complexity of understanding sex/gender or gender/sex has been expressed in publications for more than a century (Benestad & Almås, 1993; Benjamin, 1966; de Beauvoir, 1949/1976; Ehrensaft, 2017; Fausto-Sterling,

2019; Hirschfeld, 1910/1991; Hyde et al., 2018; Kessler & McKenna, 1978; van Anders, 2015). A growing amount of research supports the experience of trans people and their therapists and affirms innate sources as a basis for gender identity. There seems to be a "something" that needs confirmation and affirmation from the body as well as from the environment.

Sari van Anders' sexual configuration theory allows individual variation, involving several dimensions: appearance, behaviour, presentation, comportment, bodily features, internal sense of one's self (p. 1181) (van Anders, 2015). Janet Shibley Hyde and colleagues have explored how the idea of the "gender binary" is challenged based on neuroscience, behavioral neuroendocrinology and psychological research: "In sum, the multidimensional, complex, interactive and dynamic nature of gender/sex cannot be captured by a categorial variable, much less by a categorial variable with only two categories" (p. 15) (Hyde et al., 2018).

Non-binary gender is a concept that reflects this development. In 2020, we did a literature search, and found that *non-binary* first appeared as part of the title of a publication around 2008. This number remained stable with 0–1 publications until 2015, there was a slow increase until 2017, and it reached 176 publications in 2020 (Almås, 2020).

For some time, a third option of gender has been requested. Many countries have adopted laws to accommodate non-binary gender identities. This development has taken place since around 2009. During this period the number of applicants to gender clinics have rocketed, and many more explore gender without seeking medical assistance.

The term "transgender" was relatively new in 2002, introducing a more fluid (non-binary) approach to both sex and gender: "The formation of a transgender community denotes a newfound kinship that supplants the dichotomy of transsexual and transvestite with a concept of continuity" (Bolin, 1987; Diamond, 2002). This fluidity expresses itself in the realization that the subjective experiences of identity include somatic sex (genitals), upbringing, gender roles or sexual orientation, in different constellations.

There is no simple answer to what it is that gratifies the feeling of "being me" – but the strong feeling of *being right*, seems to be a common nominator. There is also a growing awareness among individuals, often described as *intersex*, who have had their genitals surgically "corrected"; that surgery on healthy, functioning genitals only because they do not fit into the binary model of sex and gender, has led to much unnecessary suffering. Even if many might want to live a life in congruency between subjective gender identity and sex expressed by the body, an increasing number of individuals born with ambiguous genitalia or other biological intersex-conditions ask for the right to live and be accepted as nature has made them, without surgery. The Intersex Society of North America (ISNA) is devoted to systematic change in shame, secrecy and unwanted genital surgeries for people born with anatomy that somebody decided as not standard for male or female bodies (see https://isna.org/faq/isna/mission/).

Need for Gender Affirming Treatment

Along with the development of self-affirmation and pride among trans people, an increasing number of individuals contact gender clinics for counselling and treatment (Dhejne et al., 2014). Many of these clients are challenging the binary model of gender (Ehrensaft, 2017; Ehrensaft et al., 2018; Hyde et al., 2018; Richards et al., 2016). A French study, where respondents were asked to describe their gender identity in their own words, showed a differentiation of gender identification into six categories: Woman, Man, Trans Woman, Trans Man, Trans, and Other. An increasing proportion of those who seek treatment are refraining from genital surgery. Less than one third of the sample had undergone sex reassignment surgery, one third had not made the decision yet and one third declared that they would not do it (Giami & Beaubatie, 2014).

A Norwegian study from the University of Agder, used the same questionnaire seven years later. The answers were analysed and categorized by four independent raters, resulting in a similar differentiation as the French study, but with two new categories: *non-binary* and *agender*, instead of *trans* and *other* (Almås, Bolstad et al., re-submitted for publication in 2022). A large proportion of the respondents described themselves in binary categories, as "Man" or "Woman", 45.5 per cent and 46.3 per cent respectively. In total, 16.4 per cent described themselves as trans men and 18.7 per cent as trans women. Some 25.3 per cent described themselves as non-binary. Also, 6.6 per cent of those who were assigned girls at birth and 0.8 per cent of those who were assigned boys at birth described themselves as agender.

Therapeutic assistance must be tailor made!

Individuals who experience gender incongruence represent a variety of gender identities and ask for different kinds of medical assistance. A large proportion do not ask for medical assistance at all but ask for legal and societal acceptance, first of all to be legally registered by their experienced gender identity.

A large population-based study from Sweden, asked the respondents to state agreement or disagreement to three gender related statements: "I would like hormones or surgery to be more like someone of a different sex", "I feel like someone of a different sex", and "I would like to live as or be treated as someone of a different sex". The results showed interesting differences: 0.5 per cent agreed with the first statement; 2.3 per cent agreed with the second statement; and 2.8 per cent agreed with the third statement. These results are in accordance with studies that show that gender diversity does not necessarily include a need for bodily adjustments, while for some this is paramount. In research from the University of Agder, we find that the need for treatment differed systematically with degree of binarity in their subjective experience of gender identity. The study also indicates that gender identity is better described in a dimensional model than as distinct categories.

Even if many individuals who experience gender variance have become more self-confident, have education and good jobs, many are still suffering from traumatization by not being acknowledged. Traumatization involves violent attacks, sexual assault, bullying, poverty, and imprisonment. Traumatization involves the risk for mental problems, suicidality, physical damage, both self-inflicted by use of illegal and non-monitored hormone treatment, un-ethical surgical procedures, and damage inflicted by medical doctors based on the misunderstood need to fit patients into the gender binary model.

I hope I have shown why gender identity should be regarded as a subjective experience. Most of those who seek professional assistance have been consistent in their subjective experience of gender identity for years, while others are gender explorers who may need more time to find their gendered position in a society where a variety of options are possible. Counselling and treatment must therefore be as diverse as the needs of those who seek it. Stepping down from the gate-keeping positions, counsellors and therapists must assist their clients in exploring their subjective experiences and what is right for them. A gender affirmative approach is to assist each client on the level they need. Sometimes this includes hormones, sometimes facial surgery, and to a lesser and lesser degree, genital surgery. The old idea that sexual function is not important is no longer valid.

Gender diversity is an old story – the story of binary genders is much shorter, and the non-binary model is just entering the stage, challenging us all!

Conclusion

A growing amount of research support the experience of trans-people and their therapists and affirms innate sources as a basis for gender identity. There seems to be a "something" that needs confirmation and affirmation from the body as well as from the environment. There is no simple answer to what it is that gratifies the feeling of "being me" – but the strong feeling of *being right*, seems to be a common nominator. Individuals who experience gender incongruence represent a variety of gender identities and ask for different kinds of medical assistance. A large proportion do not ask for medical assistance at all, but ask for legal and societal acceptance, first of all to be legally registered by their preferred gender identity. Counselling and treatment must therefore be as diverse as the needs of those who seek it.

About Elsa Almås

Elsa was born in Northern Norway in 1954 in a family of sailors and fishermen on one side, and forest owners and farmers on the other. Those who live by the sea are used to unpredictable luck, while those who live by the land know that they can harvest as they sow. With this inherited duality, she studied psychology, and at the same time as she found the predictable life as a clinical psychologist, she preferred the independence as a private practitioner, and adventured a career in sexology. Elsa met EE in Bergen, in 1986 where she organized a Nordic conference in sexology, and EE presented research on "heterophile transvestites". This was the beginning of a love story that is still going on. Together they started exploring the phenomenon of being trans – at that time regarded as a mental disease. Elsa and EE live in Grimstad, Norway. EE is professor emerit (not -us or -a), Elsa is still a full professor at the University of Agder, and they both have clinical practices, seeing individuals who experience gender incongruity every day.

References

Almås, E. (2020). Tokjønnsmodellen blir utfordret – rapport fra en personlig og faglig reise. *Tidsskrift for norsk Psykologforening/Journal of the Norwegian Psychological Association, 59*(9), 780–791.

Benestad, E. E. P. B. (2016). Gender belonging: Children, adolescents, adults, and the tole of the therapist. *International Journal of Narrative Therapy and Community Work, (4)*, 92–105.

Benestad, E., & Almås, E. (1993). Bekreftelsesmodell for kjønnstilhørighet. *Nordisk Sexologi, 11*(4), 209–216.

Benjamin, H. (1966). *The transsexual phenomenon*. Julian Press.

Besser, M., Carr, S., Cohen-Kettenis, P. T., Conolly, P., De Sutter, P., Diamond, M., Di Ceglie, D., Higashi, Y., Jones, L., Kruijver, F. P. M., Martin, J. L., Playdon, Z.-J., Ralph, D., Reed, T., Reid, R. C., Reiner, W. G., Swaab, D. F., Terry, T., Wilson, P. A., & Wylie, K. (2006). Atypical gender development – A review. *International Journal of Transgenderism, 9*(1), 29–44.

Bivens, R. (2017). The gender binary will not be deprogrammed: Ten years of coding gender on Facebook. *New Media & Society, 19*(6), 880–898. https://doi.org/10.1177/146144815611577

Bolin, A. (1987). *Sex and gender are different: Sexual identity and gender identity are different*. Bergin & Garvey.

Champagne, F. A. (2010). Epigenetic influence of social experience across the lifespan. *Developmental Psychobiology*. https://doi.org/10.1002/dev.20436

Clark, B. A., Veale, J. F., Townsend, M., Frohart-Dourlent, H., & Saewyc, E. M. (2019). Non-binary youth: Access to gender-affirming primary health care. *International Journal of Transgenderism*. https://doi.org/10.1080/15532739.2017.1394954

Colapinto, J. (2000). *As nature made him*. Harper-Collins Publishers.

de Beauvoir, S. (1949/1976). *Le deuxiéme sexe I, II* (Vol. *I*). Edition Gallimard.

De Block, A., & Adriaens, P. R. (2013). Pathologizing sexual deviance: A history. *Journal of Sex Research, 50*(3–4), 276–298. https://doi.org/10.1080/00224499.2012.738259

Dhejne, C., Oberg, K., Arver, S., & Landen, M. (2014, November). An analysis of all applications for sex reassignment surgery in Sweden, 1960–2010: prevalence, incidence, and regrets. *Archives of Sexual Behavior, 43*(8), 1535–1545. https://doi.org/10.1007/s10508-014-0300-8

Diamond, M. (2002). Sex and gender are different: Sexual identity and gender identity are different. *Clinical Child Psychology and Psychiatry*, *7*(3), 320–334.

Diamond, M., & Sigmundson, K. (1997). Sex reassgnment at birth. *Archives of Pediatric and Adolescent Medicine*, *151*(March), 298–304.

Dragoin, W. (1995, February 23–26). *The gynemimetic shaman. Evolutionary origins of male sexual inversion and associated talent*. International Congress on Gender, Cross Dressing and Sex Issues, California State University, Northridge

Ehrensaft, D. (2017). Gender nonconforming youth: Current perspectives. *Adolescent Health, Medicine and Therapeutics*, *19*(8), 1–18.

Ehrensaft, D., Giamattei, S. V., Storck, K., Tishelman, A. C., & Keo-Meyer, C. (2018). Prepubertal social gender transitions: What we know; what we can learn – A view from a gender affirmative lens. *International Journal of Transgenderism*, *19*(2), 251–268. https://doi.org/10.1080/15532739.2017.1414649

Fausto-Sterling, A. (2019). Gender/sex, sexual orientation, and identity are in the body: How did they get there? *The Journal of Sex Research*, 1–27. https://doi.org/10.1080/0224499.2019.151883

Foucault, M. (1976/1980). *The will to knowledge*. Vintage Books.

Freud, S. (1905/2000). *Three essays on the theory of sexuality*. The Definitive Edition, translated and revised by James Strachey. Basic Books, A Member of the Perseus Books Company.

Giami, A., & Beaubatie, E. (2014). Gender identification and sex reassignment surgery in the trans population: A survey study in France. *The Official Publication of the International Academy of Sex Research*, *43*(8), 1491–1501. https://doi.org/10.1007/s10508-014-0382-3

Hirschfeld, M. (1910/1991). *Transvestites: The erotic drive to cross dress*. Prometheus Books.

Hyde, J. S., Bigler, R. S., Joel, D., Tate, C. C., & van Anders, S. M. (2018). The future of sex and gender in psychology: Five challenges to the gender binary. *American Psychologist*. https://psycnet.apa.org/doiLanding?doi=10.1037%2Famp0000307

James, S. E., Herman, J. L., Rankin, S., Keisling, M., Mottet, L., & Ana, M. (2016). *The report of the 2015 U.S. transgender survey*.

Kessler, S., & McKenna, W. (1978). *Gender: An ethnomethodological approach*. John Wiley & Sons.

Langer, S. J. (2019). *Theorizing transgender identity for clinical practicde. A new model for understanding gender*. Jessica Kingsley Publishers.

Laqueur, T. W. (1990/2001). *Making sex. Body and gender from the Greecs to Freud*. Harvard University Press.

Money, J. (1952). *Hermaphroditism: An inquiry into the nature of a Human Paradox*. Harvard University.

Money, J., & Ehrhardt, A. (1972). *Man and woman/boy and girl*. John Hopkins University Press.

Money, J., Hampson, J. G., & Hampson, J. L. (1955). An examination of some basic sexual concepts: the evidence of human hermaphroditism. *Bulletin of the Johns Hopkins Hospita*, *97*, 301–319.

Monro, S. (2005). Beyond male and female: Poststructuralism and the spectrum of gender. *International Journal of Transgenderism*, *8*(1), 3–22. https://doi.org/10.1300/J485v08n01_02

Plato. (1987/1999/2009). *The symposium*. Penguin Books.

Plummer, K. (1991). *The making of the modern homosexual*. Rowman & Littlefield Publishers.

Rametti, G., Carillo, B., Gómez-Gil, E., Junque, C., Segovia, S., Gomez, A., & Guillamon, A. (2011). White matter microstructure in female to male transsexuals before cross-sex hormonal treatment. A diffusion tensor imaging study. *Journal of Psychiatric Research, 45*, 199–204.

Richards, C., Bouman, W. P., Seal, L., Barker, M. J., Nieder, T. O., & T'Sjoen, G. (2016). Non-binary or genderqueer genders. *International Review of Psychiatry, 28*(1), 95–102. https://doi.org/10.3109/09540261.2015.1106446

Silbersweig, D., & Loscalzo, J. (2017). Precision psychiatry meets network medicine network psychiatry. *JAMA Psychiatry, 74*(7), 665–666.

van Anders, S. M. (2015). Beyond sexual orientation: Integrating gender/sex and diverse sexualities via sexual configuration theory. *Archives of Sexual Behavior, 44*, 1177–1213.

von Krafft-Ebing, R. (1997). *Psychopathia sexualis*. The Case Histories. Velvet.

Zhou, J., Hofman, M. A., Gooren, L. J. G., & Swaab, D. F. (1995). A sex difference in the human brain and its relation to transsexuality. *Nature, 378*(November 1995), 68–70.

Chapter 3

Holding Uncertainty So That It Can Be Thought About

Relational Gestalt Therapy with Gender Creative Children

Dominic Hosemans

Despite being an extremely important topic in the context of mental health, the literature describing the therapeutic work with 'gender creative' (Ehrensaft, 2017) individuals is extremely sparse. Recently, some relational gestalt therapists have discussed work with gender creative adults, for instance, Bennett (2010), Johnson (2014), and Vikram Kolmannskog (2014); however, no attention has been directed towards work with gender creative children in context of relational gestalt therapy. The latter provides a very unique perspective in terms of working with gender creative children owing to its focus on contacting processes and the development of awareness. Gender creative children often come to counselling with a strong sense of guilt and shame for their internal experience, which is very often inconsistent with their outward appearance. Such an internalised sense of an 'unacceptable self' often manifests as intense anxiety, anger or withdrawal as a result of not wanting to be in contact with their own internal world due to not fitting the predefined categories of gender experience. By the gestalt therapist developing a sense of curiosity and demonstrating the capacity to tolerate and hold the child's uncertain and chaotic internal worlds, it becomes possible to begin experiencing what feels intolerable and thus start developing awareness regarding the child's internal experience. Essentially, the child's internal experience can only be thought about if it can be tolerated. The capacity to tolerate such experience occurs within an inter-subjective paradigm.

Cultivating Uncertainty

The most important therapeutic principle for working with gender creative children is the capacity to sit with a large degree of uncertainty and simultaneously tolerating the anxiety that this may manifest within the therapist. Such a capacity to 'just sit with' entails being in the 'dark' with the child's internal world until what is meant to become figural is illuminated. Without the process of staying in the dark regarding what will arise, the person of the child is consequently not met. This means that information on the referral as well as discussions with the child's parents need to be bracketed and yet simultaneously held in mind. Doing psychotherapeutic work with children is

DOI: 10.4324/9781003335344-3

more of an art, with the art being defined by balancing the tension between the certainty of the therapist's professional experience and psychological theories with the uncertainty of what may arise in the here-and-now of the experiential process.

Anxiety is a consequence of uncertainty, which can very quickly evolve into a sense of panic over not knowing what to do at any given moment in the therapeutic setting; however, such moments just require space for the not-yet-formed to become figural. Doing something in reactance to the therapist's need to be effective or to see changes, in and of itself, detracts from the therapist's capacity to 'just be with' the individual in any way that the child needs at that very moment; which often changes throughout the therapeutic process. Therapy with children needs to be perceived as a fluid process, which constantly moves and paradoxically is thematically the same. As soon as the therapist defines what it is the child needs or what needs to be worked on, the child is consequently no longer invited to be in contact, but rather the child changes in order to become what is expected of them. Thus, cutting off any capacity for relationality. This is often a difficult balance, especially with children, as they typically present to therapy with someone who is expecting to see tangible and quantifiable changes.

Nonetheless, uncertainty or 'worlding' (Spinelli, 2007) is a necessary but not sufficient process for growth of the individual. The experience of 'worlding' needs to additionally be accommodated and adapted within one's 'worldview', in which there is oscillation between the two, and, by extension oscillation from certainty to uncertainty. Too much uncertainty equates to feeling overwhelmed, whereas not enough uncertainty transforms one's ideas into a very fixed perception or gestalt of the world. Thus, there is a constant balance, especially within the therapeutic space, of allowing just enough uncertainty, but being able to connect the experience of 'worlding' to the client's perception of the world, with each experience of 'worlding' facilitating to extend the child's horizon of awareness. According to a number of existentialists (for a review, see Crowell, 2017), this balance is essentially the tension of existence. Growth thus only occurs by virtue of being able to sit with the tension between certainty and uncertainty. A child's capacity grows very rapidly due to their experience of the world being not-yet-formed in cognition and yet this is contrasted with a world in which they are situated that appears to perpetuate certainty in ideas, such as ideas regarding gender and its expression.

Working with children, and this is very true with issues associated with gender creativity, is more an embodied process rather than a cognitive one. To ask a child why they did something, there is no ability for them to answer, as their experience of the world is an embodied one. As such, there is no logical reasoning as to why something is, it was just felt to be, and the experience is not-yet-formed in cognition. Current mainstream models of psychotherapy do an injustice to the understanding of a child's internal world. There is a pervasive belief that there is a primacy of cognition. Yet, such an understanding is based on Descartes' (1996) cogito argument, where one is a thinking being with a body, rather than an embodied being with a thinking mind. Working with children, one needs to consider the primacy of affect (McGilchrist, 2009) and embodiment, which in turn is thought about in order to make sense of and develop an understanding. Cognition needs to be of something, which invariably, for children, is their embodied sense of the world.

Following Piaget's (Piaget & Inhelder, 2000) insights about child development, children do not yet have the cognitive capacity to make sense of their embodied experience of the world. Children essentially need an external mind to hold, or sense, their internal world and provide thought and words around their experience. For example, a child being quite destructive with some toys, rather than trying to augment the form of play, the therapist helps the child reflect of their destructiveness, by reflecting, "you are so angry right now, and it is very important that you show me how angry you are". Not only does this have the effect of helping the child make sense of their internal world, it also demonstrates to the child that you are able to tolerate these more unnameable parts of themselves.

Thus, prior to helping a child make sense of their internal world, especially their relationship with gender, it is absolutely essential that a child is able to tolerate their internal world. If one is unable to tolerate what is happening within their embodied experience of the world, there are other psychological mechanisms at play, such as avoidance, deflection, or projection. These psychological mechanisms facilitate in making one's experience of the world more of a cognitive process rather than an embodied one. As already indicated, such a perception is a fallacy, and results in an experience, of what Sartre (2007) would call, 'bad faith'. Fundamentally, when one is not being authentic to one's current phenomenological experience, as such, one is unable to make sense of something that is not being truly experienced.

Systemic Certainty as Cause of Distress

Paul was a eight-year-old boy who was starting to identify as a girl. Paul preferred the personal pronoun 'he' and to still be called by his birth name. However, he would sometimes come to our sessions in a very extravagant princess dress with his nails all painted to match. My impression of Paul was that he was very confident within himself but really craved the acceptance of others, which was not necessarily forthcoming due to his difficult home-life situation. At the time of his birth, Paul's mother was already in her early to mid-forties, and he was a baby whom she desperately wanted at the protest of her boyfriend. In infancy, Paul's mother reported that his father was often very abusive to both of them; with the Department of Human Services being notified a number of times. Paul's mother was courageous enough to leave her partner prior to Paul's first birthday, but the difficulties within the family system continued, with Paul's father deciding when he wanted to see Paul on a very sporadic basis.

From our first session together, it was clear that Paul wanted to do the therapeutic work. Upon entering my office, Paul looked around the room, and then asked if we could play cafes. I had asked Paul what this would look like, and he had indicated that he wanted to cook something for me to eat. For a good ten minutes of our first meeting together, he worked very hard in the play kitchenette area of my office making sure that he was able to look after me. This was very important to Paul; he was essentially making sure that he developed a good relational foundation with me in order to be able to journey together through the difficult times ahead. After my imaginary hunger was abated, he had asked me, in turn, to step into his kitchen and make him something to eat. Paul was very specific in regards to what he wanted cooked for him, a large nutritious meal, seemingly suggesting that from the therapeutic space, he wanted to be well looked after and nurtured – something that he lacked and craved. This was one of the many times that he wanted to engage in such play in order to have the sense that he was held within the therapeutic space.

The creative relational play formed the foundations for our discussions, which were very difficult for Paul. However, we had already securely developed the 'in-between' space as nurturing and mutually protective. At times, rather than playing, he would sit on the couch and talk for the entire session. His discussions would range from what was happening at school, his experience at home, what he was currently reading and immersed in, as well as his experience of being in his body, especially in terms of a body he often felt was not his. His descriptions of his body were quite mixed, not knowing at times if he were in actuality a boy or if he were a girl. His mother thought that his experience was just a phase that he was going through, understanding but at the same time dismissive of his experience. His father's reaction was a different story altogether.

After approximately our fifteenth session together, Paul told his father that he was unsure if he identified as a boy or girl. The session thereafter was the most difficult session we ever had together, and in retrospect, I can see how it was so important for Paul to initially establish a strong foundation between us. He essentially needed a place where his rage would be welcomed without needing him to react in any other way. This particular session was the essence of being able to tolerate 'what is', even if the child is unable to tolerate such things. Already on our way into my office I could see that he was struggling on this particular day. He wiped some tears from his eyes, hitting the wall of the hallway on our way into my office. He was the embodiment of rage.

As soon as he entered my office, all the things that we had built together, he began to destroy. He said that he does not care about anything; he hated everything; that he was no good; that there was something inherently wrong with him; and that he did not want to live anymore. He started with the play kitchenette area, and began to smash everything to the ground. All the good that we had built together in the therapy room, he had split from it and made it mean nothing. From the kitchenette area, Paul began to destroy many of the other toys in the room. He was so immensely angry, regardless of what I had reflected to him, he continued to destroy everything good that he had built up in the therapeutic space. Following the ideas of Kline (Segal, 1982), he had 'split' from all that was good in his life. As gestalt therapy grew out of, and is the flourishing, of psychoanalytic thinking, relational gestalt therapy aims to transcend such 'splits' in thinking in order to allow the individual to experience themselves as a 'whole person'.

Such intense uncontained reactions typically occur within children due to not being able to tolerate an embodied experience, with the internalised reaction an attempt to rid oneself of the intolerable embodiment. By the end of the session, the entire room was in disarray, with toys thrown all across the floor. Paul was on the couch crying inconsolably, unable to catch his breath. In short bursts of words, punctuated with the heaving of his lungs, he told me that his father said he never wanted to see him again. Paul was deeply devastated. His devastation was impossible to contain within himself. Paul indicated that he felt that he was inherently bad for whom he was, and therefore not deserving of any good within his life. In reaction to this embodied experience, Paul attempted to get rid of the therapeutic foundations that we had built together. My sense was that he was also expecting me to reject him and he was trying to give me good reason to. However, we just stayed with his anger until it passed, demonstrating to him that I have the capacity to tolerate his anger, which he then perceived and began to internalise my capacity to tolerate within our inter-subjective paradigm. The session subsequent to Paul's experienced rage, Paul was quite tentative in coming back into my office, but when he did, not a word was spoken. He went straight to the kitchenette area and began to make me something nutritious to eat, this time recounting even more details of all the things he needed to do in order to cook his recipe. By being able to tolerate such 'splits' in thinking, Paul was able to hold onto the good things within his mind and the world.

'Living through' Paul's rage alongside him, helped Paul to internalise the capacity to tolerate such difficult feelings. The very small amount of literature on working with children in a relational gestalt context, essentially suggests the co-construction of the 'in-between' space as well as providing the therapist particular activities in which the child is invited to partake (for instance, see: Blom, 2004; Oaklander, 2007). However, such strategies have the consequence of shutting down uncertainty and potentially help the therapist more than the child in the moment (Bugental, 1981). Rather, the way I worked with Paul was very organic, allowing him to construct the 'in-between space' according to what he needed from the therapy. Children, and in particular gender creative children, already have a sense of what they want to work on (Landreth, 2012), but such a sense exists within their not-yet-formed internal life-world. The therapist's role then is primarily to provide that space, suspended in uncertainty, in order for the not-yet-formed to become figural.

There is no universal way of 'being' with others in their distress. A therapist essentially needs to tune into the 'in-between' space and understand how it is that the client is using the space in order to show the therapist what it is that they experience at a phenomenological level (Grossmark, 2018). Rather than the co-construction of the 'in-between' space, especially when working with children and more so with gender creative children, fundamental to the work of the therapist is to allow the 'in-between' space to be projected into from the child's psyche, so that the therapist is able to understand, make sense of, and feedback what it is that is happening for the child on an embodied level. The therapist then acts as a 'container' (Winnicott, 1960) of the child's projections, only feeding back to the child what they are essentially able to take back in. There is an art to such balancing, as the therapist may understand certain aspects of the child's phenomenological experience early on in the therapeutic process, but there is insufficient ground or support within the field for the child to appropriately assimilate such information.

Certainty as a Defence against Anxiety

The world is a very uncertain place and how one protects against such uncertainty is through adopting particular belief systems that provide a sense of certainty, such as mainstream cultural ideas, religious systems of thought, political ideologies. Regardless of what the individual adheres to, the underlying essence is the same – a defence against the anxiety of uncertainty. As an extension of this idea, generally people develop a fixed conceptualisation of self rather than felt-sense of self that changes according to their interaction with the wider field. In this way the individual cannot be considered as separate from the field in which they are situated in the context of understanding themselves. For instance, the language one uses, the objects of consciousness, the surrounding environment that one attends to, are all aspects of the field – the field flows through one continuously in a fluid motion. Just like the field, a fixed definition cannot suffice to describe an individual. Such a need for certainty in order to alleviate anxiety also infiltrates through society's ideas regarding gender. Mainstream ideas conceptualise an individual as either a male or female, without any uncertainty of the space between. Within an inter-subjective context, those who defend against uncertainty end up projecting their anxiety onto those who do not fit neatly within the ascribed categories of existence. The experience of anxiety that is perpetuated by a system that seeks certainty, is especially felt by children who are gender creative.

For instance, Timothy ascribed to the personal pronouns of 'their' or 'they' as Timothy did not identify specifically with either gender but actually expressed themselves as either male or female depending on the situation and how they were feeling within the moment. Rather than switching from one to the other, Timothy expressed elements of both genders to different degrees depending upon the context. Timothy was a ten-year old born male who had initially presented for counselling with their mother due to feeling uncertain about how they were expressing themselves, looking essentially to find a sense of certainty, as either being male or female. Timothy reported that the feeling of not knowing, or uncertainty, was the cause of their anxiety. Timothy's perception of themselves was primarily based on a cultural climate that wished to translate all experience into particular categories without the greyness that exists within the fertile void. Thus, due to not fitting perfectly within such a category, Timothy felt incredibly anxious that there was something inherently wrong with them.

When working with gender creativity, within the context of the phenomenological field, it is not sufficient to develop awareness of what is occurring and how one is relating to the wider field. Such a stance essentially situates the phenomenological field as fixed and unchangeable. Rather, within the context of children, relational gestalt therapy also needs to work towards helping the individuals to consider changing the wider phenomenological field in order to facilitate the conditions for their optimal growth and flourishing and to live, as Sartre would say, in good faith. For instance, Timothy would indicate that they felt very uncomfortable and unable to learn during the day at school as they felt like they were wearing the wrong uniform and therefore felt isolated and out of place. Oftentimes, Timothy would wake up feeling more feminine and wanting to express this by virtue of wearing tights and a dress, which they reported to accompany a feeling of being free and authentic. However, the phenomenological field in which Timothy was situated still retained a gender binary policy around school uniforms. This issue needed to be discussed with the school in order to be able to support Timothy's mental health within the school environment.

It is even more evident than with adult clients that children exist within an interconnected field, thus the interventions also need to take into account the structure of the field for any gender creative child. Thus, work with gender creative children occurs not only within the therapeutic session, but also impacting the phenomenological field in which they are situated. Working with the family dynamic as well as advocacy in the client's lived-world is essential in order to support the therapeutic work. In fact, without facilitating to effect change in the child's wider phenomenological field, the therapeutic work has very little impact. This is essentially because children do not have the power within their own lives to change how they are responded to and treated within the environment. Considering the therapist sees the child for potentially one hour per week, whereas the child is always situated within the family dynamic, the child's family really hold the key in being able to support the child's mental health.

Considerations for Working with Gender Creative Children

As previously discussed, the therapist needs to remain open and receptive to how the gender creative child constructs the 'in-between' space in a way that is beneficial to their growth and development. A substantial and significant part of being open and receptive is the capacity to remain uncertain and to tolerate such an experience without the need to close down on a sense of certainty in order to alleviate the therapist's anxiety of 'not knowing'. In this way, the therapist is able to hold what is projected into the 'in-between' space, make sense of it, and give it back in a way that can be assimilated. As soon as the therapist is looking for a sense of certainty, such as linking back the child's experience to their relevant professional experience or to a particular theory, the felt-sense of the 'in-between' space is lost, with all that is reflected back to the child instead a general abstraction that is now removed from any degree of here-and-now relationality. By being able to 'sit with' and tolerate uncertainty, the therapist is reflecting their capacity to stay with the child's distress. In turn, within the relational dynamic, the child introjects the thera-pist's capacity to 'sit with' what is.

Although words are very important, as they contain a particular meaning depending upon the context, it would not have mattered as much what was said between Timothy or Paul and myself. Essentially, I was able to stay with the sense of uncertainty, whilst using this experience as the driver as to where our conversation was destined. It was then possible to follow as closely as possible the phenomenological experience of the client within the here-and-now with the intent of not only helping them to become more aware of what occurs on the horizon of their awareness, but also being an external mind that can help them make sense of their experience. The latter processes essentially rest upon the capacity to tolerate internal experience – as only what can be tolerated can be thought about. Furthermore, each child needed me to be a different type of therapist within the therapeutic space. This was expressed within their construction of the 'in-between' space, thus required me to patiently wait 'in the dark' to determine how they needed to arrange the ground of experience in order to allow their internal world to be seen.

According to Stolorow, Brandchaft and Atwood (1987), the mind is essen-tially an inter-subjective phenomenon. There is no coming to mind without at first being in relationship. Paradoxically, an individual mind can only come into being by virtue of relating with another mind. Winnicott (1960) initially indicated that there is no such thing as a baby, meaning that the baby only exists through relating with their primary caregiver. From the idea of the mind being an inter-subjective phenomenon, it is clear that psychological distress, rather than isolated within one's mind, occurs within relationship. An individual's distress primarily arises through relationship, such as how one relates to the world and whether or not the world relates back in a way that is open and receptive to whom they perceive themselves to be. As what happens for a number of gender creative children, if in the context of an important relationship, it is reflected back to the child that they are not accepted for who they are, this idea is introjected and therefore a cause of considerable distress. But the distress is more a systemic issue, and needs to be held by those around them in order to be tolerated and therefore thought about.

About Dominic Hosemans, PhD

Dr Dominic Hosemans is a registered counselling psychologist working in private practice. Dominic has been interested in gestalt therapeutic ideas since completing a number of years of study in philosophy prior to studying psychology. He completed his PhD on the phenomenological experience of equanimity within meditation. Prior to commencing official training in gestalt therapy with gestalt Therapy Australia, Dominic was a lecturer at Monash University on statistics and research design. He additionally was a senior supervisor for a number of Honours and Masters projects concerning scale development.

References

Bennett, J. L. (2010). "Inocencia": Case Study of a Transgender Woman without Gender Dysphoria Preparing for Gender Reassignment Surgery. *British Gestalt Journal, 19*(2), 16–27.

Blom, R. (2004). *The Handbook of Gestalt Play Therapy: Practical Guidelines for Child Therapists*. London, UK: Jessica Kingsley Publishers.

Bugental, J. F. T. (1981). *The Search for Authenticity: An Existential-Analytic Approach to Psychotherapy*. New York, NY: Irvington.

Crowell, S. (2017). Existentialism. In E. N. Zalta (Ed.), *The Stanford Encyclopedia of Philosophy*. Retrieved from https://plato.stanford.edu/archives/win2017/entries/existentialism/

Descartes, R. (1996). *Meditations on First Philosophy*. (J. Cottingham, Ed.). Cambridge, UK: Cambridge University Press.

Ehrensaft, D. (2017). *The Gender Creative Child*. New York, NY: The Experiment LLC.

Grossmark, R. (2018). *The Unobtrusive Relational Analyst: Exporations in Psychoanalytic Companioning*. New York, NY: Routledge.

Johnson, R. A. E. (2014). Contacting Gender. *Gestalt Review, 18*(3), 207–225.

Kolmannskog, V. (2014). Gestalt Approaches to Gender Identity Issues: A Case Study of a Transgender Therapy Group in Oslo. *Gestalt Review, 18*(3), 244–260. Retrieved from http://www.jstor.org/stable/10.5325/gestaltreview.18.3.0244

Landreth, G. L. (2012). *Play Therapy: The Art of the Relationship* (3rd ed.). New York, NY: Routledge.

McGilchrist, I. (2009). *The Master and his Emissary: The Divided Brain and the Making of the Western World*. London: Yale University Press.

Oaklander, V. (2007). *Windows to Our Children: A Gestalt Therapy Approach to Children and Adolescents*. Goulsboro, Maine: Gestalt Journal Press.

Piaget, J., & Inhelder, B. (2000). *The Psychology of the Child*. New York, NY: Basic Books.

Sartre, J.-P. (2007). *Existentialism is a Humanism*. New Haven: Yale University Press.

Segal, H. (1982). *Introduction to the Work of Melanie Klein*. London, UK: The Hogarth Press and the Institute of Psychoanalysis.

Spinelli, E. (2007). *Practising Existential Psychotherapy: The Relational World*. California: SAGE Publications Inc.

Stolorow, R. D., Brandchaft, B., & Atwood, G. E. (1987). *Psychoanalytic Treatment: An Intersubjective Approach*. El Dorado Hills, CA: Analytic Press.

Winnicott, D. W. (1960). The Theory of the Parent–Infant Relationship. *International Journal of Psycho-Analysis*, *41*, 585–595.

Chapter 4

The Drag and Queer Years as a Means of Developing a Therapeutic Self

Bringing Street Work in the Office

Parvy Palmou

The Drag and Queer Years as a Means of Developing a Therapeutic Self

My first contact with the trans community was at Koukles Club, a drag show club in Sygrou Avenue, Athens. As a 19-year-old genderqueer bisexual and undergraduate psychology student, I made my first steps at Koukles as a DJ. While relishing this house of dance and feathers at first, I soon became acquainted with the violence, racism, and exclusion our community faces. In the street, the clients were often violent and the beatings were nothing short of uncommon, leaving my friends abused and in life-threatening situations every night near the club. Standing on the street, out in the cold, they earned their living the hard way. I remember on one occasion, clients passing by with their cars throwing fruits filled with razors at them with the intention to hurt them. It was this incident, on that day, which urged me to the decision to work with this population, the community I am also part of, the LGBTQIA community, as soon as I finished my studies and became a psychotherapist. My goal became to help trans people be included in society and to help society overcome transphobia. To help them handle the impact on their lives and bodies while focusing on depathologization. So, as soon as I concluded my BA and MA back in 2010, I started working as psychotherapist at the Greek Transgender Support Association (GTSA). To this day, I proudly support the Association as the Head of the Department of Health for Trans and Intersex Families.

Bringing Street Work Inside the Office

Most of the members of the association are trans women sex workers with a traumatic background. One of them characteristically mentioned to me once "I was raised in an orphanage so when I ended up in jail, it did not feel any different; it felt like home to me." I brought myself into therapy and relied on gestalt to include my own life and experiences. The self-disclosure of my own LGBTQIA status was a pivotal point in developing rapport and therapeutic alliance. Using relational gestalt practices and my own experience as a non-binary, genderqueer, bisexual person helped me establish an authentic

DOI: 10.4324/9781003335344-4

contact and a broad understanding of gender and sexuality issues. My clinical background was always helpful but not enough to support me in this new role; gestalt-based self-revelation and authenticity were more relationship and contact-oriented. Gender incongruence was happening in the body, abuse was happening in the body, so that was where our work during therapy was focused and where gestalt was incorporated. During our sessions, I also came to realize the importance of language in our communication and I felt the need to bring into the office the slang that trans people use in the street, which in Greek is called "Kaliarda". Alongside therapy, my job was also to inform them about STDs and HIV, and provide information about free testing and the effects of hormonal treatment on HIV medication. On many occasions, after our sessions, trans sex workers left the Association with a protection kit, which is usually given to street workers by health organizations. My role as a psychotherapist was not enough; I had to assume the role of a health instructor, co-worker, fellow queer, and most importantly a person that speaks the same language. These multiple roles required continuous therapy and supervision, and my yearly participation in Transgender Europe and ILGA Europe trainings and congresses as well as trainings in LGBTQIA health conducted by the Council of Europe. Since 2018, I also assumed the role of consultant in the Interdisciplinary Commission for the Legal Gender Recognition and Access to Health of Trans Teenagers at the Greek Ministry of Health.

LGBTQIA Affirmative Gestalt Therapy

I started developing my approach, a combination of gestalt therapy and LGBTQIA affirmative therapy, driven from the above-described experiences back in 2012 and I have since presented it to many universities in Athens and Thessaloniki, e.g. the Hellenic Psychoanalytic Society, the Hellenic Focusing Center, the Air Force General Hospital, the Greek Sexology Institute, and the University of the Aegean, which included this training as a 600-hour course. This particular course was developed together with my co-trainer, Anna Apergi, a trans woman, and it constitutes the first of its kind for Greece.

The development of the approach is still ongoing. However, in the following sections, I will make an effort to describe the seven main principles on which the LGBTQIA affirmative gestalt therapy is based.

In order to do so, I would like to introduce a specific case study in order to support further understanding of the flow of therapy in the various stages. I feel that following the process of a specific client through the various stages will be helpful for the reader.

Case Presentation

General information: All the case information is made public and available following the informed consent of the person, who for the purposes of this presentation will be nicknamed Nico. So, Nico first approached me for therapy in 2011. Nico was referred to me from the Greek Transgender Support Association where they had joined as a member. They were 45 years old, originally from a small town and residing in Athens. Nico was divorced twice, with one daughter aged 17 years old from the first marriage, and a 4-year-old boy from the second marriage. They worked as a personal assistant. They came to therapy after interrupting the treatment with a psychiatrist because they did not feel met by the treatment provided (too directive and judgemental). They wanted to be supported by an expert in case they decided to proceed to transition.

The main therapeutic goals (co-created in the first sessions) were:

1   Understanding their gender identity.
2   Support during transition (in case they made that decision).
3   Support – coming out – disclosure of gender identity and sexual orientation to the social environment and family.
4   Exploring the possibility of coming out – disclosing their identity to the children (fear of rejection and exclusion).
5   Fear of social, economic exclusion from society after the transition.
6   Practical information on transition-hormone treatment and change of legal documents etc.

Background and preliminary questions

- On the question 'what you would like to achieve from therapy', they replied 'mental and spiritual peacefulness, increase of self-acceptance, and understanding'.
- On the question 'do you feel sadness or depression', they answered 'yes, I have been feeling depressed for the last 2 years that my gender dysphoria intensified'.
- There is no history of psychiatric diagnoses in them and their family; they only reported that their mother is generally anxious.

Using Gender-Neutral Language and Correct Pronouns

Therapy commences from the first call, thus a therapist working with this population has to be conscious and inclusive. The use of gender-neutral language is very important until the client provides us with information about the gender identity. Some of the clients are not yet ready – not even after months of therapy – so the use of this language is of great importance in order to help the client feel comfortable, accepted and safe. We cannot assume a person's gender identity by their voice on the phone, their appearance in the room, or any other external characteristic. We know from statistics that intersex people are born with the same frequency as people with red hair, whilst in many countries the statistics are incomplete due to the "normalization" operations performed at a young age so that the person does not even know that they were born intersex. Some trans people do not identify with the gender attributed to them at birth and they are non-binary, while some others identify as genderqueer. Bearing that in mind, a person specializing in mental health needs to be aware of the high probability that a gender non-confirming person will pick up the phone or even walk through the office door, as these incidents are not so rare. Our biases can be extremely transphobic and offensive in terms of terminology and/or slang. Respect of pronouns and neutral language is the first step to an inclusive gender diversity affirmative gestalt therapy.

When Nico first visited me, for example, they mentioned "I don't know yet how I want you to refer to me (meaning the pronouns she/he/they). I don't know yet if I will proceed to the transition." Nico was unaware of their gender incongruence realising that "something was wrong", but did not know what. They felt different, but did not know in what respect until about the age of 42 when they began to understand what was happening. Therapy started in the confusion phase and that's why the gender-neutral language in therapy is very important until the person can self-identify. It should be noted at this point that at the beginning of treatment, Nico began with an appearance considered by society to be highly masculine, i.e. tall, with big shoulders, short hair, and a heavy voice. The use of gender-neutral language ceased when they chose the name (Nico) and pronoun (she/her) that she would like me to use.

Working with Internalized Transphobia

Through my work I came to consider a person's assigned gender as an introjection – in gestalt terms. Initially, the role of an introjection is to violently interrupt the natural flow of the body. Caregivers tend to unconsciously inculcate introjections, which very often conflict with the natural flow of the person at all levels. In sexual orientation and gender identity in particular, the assigned gender or assigned sexuality is never assimilated by the body since it is perceived as a foreign object. So, depending on the resilience of the person, there will be an internal conflict between the real gender and the heteronormative introjection of the idea created by the gender binary. This internal conflict is where internalized transphobia, hatred of self, hatred of body, feeling of gender incongruence derive from. Of course, not all LGBTQIA people go through this stage. Depending on their resilience and the support of the environment, some of us have worked through these challenges at a very early stage or we have not and will not experience them at all.

In our first months of therapy, although we were making a lot of progress, Nico had a huge difficulty in understanding, identifying, and working with the polarities that were so complex and confusing for her. For years, she had been playing the role of the "man" and the father. In a way she had blocked her ability to come in contact with her authentic self, she was fragmented, and the fragments were fixed gestalts about her gender, appearance, and place in society. These fixed gestalts did not provide the space for the new form to emerge and for her to view herself as a whole. I created an exercise. We started with focusing on the body and she identified the polarity in the neck and chest as a burden. I asked her to give a voice to the burden and she replied that the neck part was the "female side" that it was connected to calmness and peace. She felt a calming feeling describing this, and the point of the chest, which was the "male" side connected to programming and enthusiasm. She identified a split as she could not feel female and enthusiastic or being in charge and she could not be male and feel calm. She could not feel whole. I asked her to draw what she had seen, and she created the image below. Using the skills from relational art therapy that I was trained in, we worked on this sketch for 4 sessions doing bodywork, chair work, and relational gestalt. When Nico participated in my Ψ-Architecture workshop using a practice from the Theatre of the Oppressed (see Section 4), she enacted her polarity in the group and one group member was asked to play her mirror. During the feedback, we identified that her two polarities started to support each other, learned to work together, and were now increasingly integrated in the organism.

Working with Gender Identity and Sexual Orientation Introjections

Based on my experience, clients approach me at a stage where they have identified some kind of an internal conflict. As a 45-year-old trans person, Nico told me at the beginning "I am too masculine, I have huge hands, huge shoulders, I will never be the woman I want to be even after transition, I will be

POLARITY Ψ-ARCHITECTURE

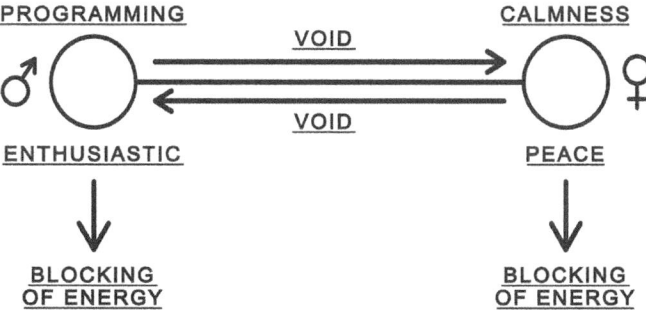

Figure 4.1 The following is a Ψ-Architecture exercise based on focusing techniques. The client focuses on the body and discovers a polarity (male vs female) that creates an internal imbalance and conflict. On the left side of the polarity, the "male" side. The client identifies the ability of being able to program their everyday life, be in control and have enthusiastic energy but lacks calmness and peace which creates a blocking of somatic energy focused on the chest. The client reports a split, they can either be on the one side of the polarity or the other. There is no balance, no equilibrium, and the movement between the two poles creates a void that is related to fear of transition from male to female introjected qualities.

a monster; whatever I do is hopeless!" She also expressed her confusion in other comments like "I am a trans woman and I am attracted to women, is this possible. Maybe there is something wrong with me!" Often, the conflict is between body and gender expression. Nico was so confused at first that she believed that she had a psychiatric condition, such as Paranoia or OCD, or Dissociative Disorder.

Gestalt experimental exercises for deconstructing introjections using Ψ-Architecture (example of the polarity of gender incongruence drawing)

Using Methods of Expression and Movement Borrowed and Adjusted from the Theatre of the Oppressed

During my training in 2015, I came across the Theatre of the Oppressed, in the Czech Republic. I took a 15-day course in a retreat in the mountains, resulting in a play about transphobia that we presented in Brno. I assumed the roles of director and actress in that play, which you can see here: www.facebook.com/parvy.paradoxia/videos/483456385147864.

During this training, it came to my attention that some of the practices would be useful and should be integrated in my work and combined with my usual gestalt practices, e.g. the *de-mechanization exercises*. Augusto Boal, creator of the Theatre of the Oppressed, used a set of exercises to reduce the mechanization of the body, so it could be more receptive to change. These exercises are very simple, e.g. walking backwards; when you hear sit, you jump; when you hear run, you stop; and a combination of all these before working with the body individually, or in a group. My idea was that if the assigned gender is an introjection – a mechanization of society – then these exercises would be extremely effective. And they are.

Nico also participated in group therapy sessions I was leading in GTSA. In these settings I used almost all exercises by Augusto Boal with the trans and gender non-confirming group.

Using the Stages of Coming Out

Gender non-confirming people usually come for therapy when they discover a polarity or when an internal conflict between their two sides (gender identity and body image) has begun within the self. Inevitably, this leads to a conflict with the environment, since every unresolved conflict within the person will become interpersonal in the future.

Based on the stages of coming out created by Cass (1979), the first stage that most LGBTQIA experience is the confusion of identity.

Cass (1979) General Theory

Stage 1   Identity confusion
Stage 2   Identity comparison

Stage 3   Identity tolerance
Stage 4   Identity acceptance
Stage 5   Identity pride
Stage 6   Identity synthesis

Although Cass created this model for homosexuals, I empirically concluded that trans people also go through similar stages. In the confusion of identity stage, a "sense of incongruence" develops, i.e. a conflict between their perception of themselves as trans and the realization of thoughts and feelings of incongruence. This is when trans and gender non-confirming people usually seek therapy. The therapist should be aware of the stage they are in and have a deep understanding of what this stage means to the person, so that the therapist can meet them where they are.

In the first steps of therapy (about six months), Nico started to feel extremely interested in learning more about the community. Except GTSA, where she was already a member, she was engaged in a lesbian organization, and an organization of LGBTQIA families, where she made a lot of friends and found support. At this point, her social transition included changing her social life so she could fit in. She did not come out in her work environment at that point.

After about eight months of therapy she took the decision to start on stable hormone administration. My therapeutic style is non-directive and following previous research I never engage in gatekeeping, i.e. suggesting to a trans person not to do any intervention on their body, except if there is a serious medical or mental threat. My work is affirming and supporting, based solely on self-determination. I always make sure that any intervention on the body – such as hormones or surgeries – is done following informed consent on health risks, statistics, and good practices. All the decisions are taken by the persons themselves, during therapy, with me fully respecting their bodily autonomy and supporting their decisions.

I often get asked how some people perceive their gender identity or sexual orientation too early or –apparently – too late in their lives. I believe that in this kind of self-perception introjections play a significant role. When these introjections are strong, the person perceives and comes into contact with their authentic self later in life.

Nico, was over 40 years old when she first realized that incongruence. And one of her major concerns was her coming out with her transgender identity to her children aged 4 and 17. She mentioned to me "I'm not afraid of surgery as much as I'm afraid of losing my children, they are the most important thing in my life." Provision of psychoeducational material on the trans identity for the two mothers and their 17-year-old daughter was the first step. The psychoeducation to the four-year-old child who is now ten continues slowly and steadily until today with a very positive outcome.

Since my training and certification do not involve working with children, the children were not involved in therapy. My work was focused on providing the steps and good practices for Nico to work with her children. We found a LGBTQIA friendly child psychiatrist–psychotherapist to support the children and the mothers and I was always available for any question they had. The children reacted very positively. Unfortunately, this is not always the case for trans parents. Still, we know from experience and research that if the parents and the environment is accepting, and there is adequate psychoeducation and support from therapists, the children can be very supportive of the parent's identity; in some cases, even more than adults. The older daughter is now an LGBTQIA ally and advocate.

Conclusion

Regarding Nico and her bodily condition, at the end of 2014 and after 2.5 years of hormone administration as provided for by WPATH good practices, I accompanied Nico to Serbia where she received her gender confirmation surgery at a specialist clinic. I provided psychological support throughout and after the surgery. We continued supportive therapy for eight months after surgery showing significant improvement at all levels until discontinuation of treatment.

One year after our last session together, I usually ask clients to write something about the impact of therapy on their lives. Nico stated I now live an authentic fulfilled and happy life, I accept myself and my children and family supports me. I guess now my life is very normal, with normal problems. The issue of gender belongs in the past for me. She is currently the proud owner of a restaurant in Athens, Greece.

About Parvy Palmou

Parvy Palmou received her MA in Clinical Psychology from the University of Indianapolis in 2007. She is an accredited gestalt therapist, working privately in Athens Greece. For the last 11 years she has been Head of the Department of Health for Trans and Intersex Families at the Greek Transgender Support Association where she practises gestalt therapy with transgender, intersex, and non-binary people. She is an international trainer and a regular columnist in various newspapers, magazines, and websites and has achieved several publications. Currently she is a visiting professor at the University of the Aegean for the LGBTQI+ Gestalt Affirmative Counseling Program and a PhD candidate at the University of Bolton performing research on trans health and wellbeing. You can contact Parvy Palmou at palmoup@hotmail.com.

Bibliography

Alessi, E. J., & Martin, J. I. (2017). Intersection of trauma and identity. In K. L. Eckstrand & J. Potter (Eds), *Trauma, resilience, and health promotion in LGBT patients* (pp. 3–14). Cham, Switzerland: Springer. https://doi.org/10. 1007/978-3-319-54509-7_1

Augusto Boal's 'Theatre of the Oppressed'. (2003). Retrieved 1 September 2021, from https://news.harvard.edu/gazette/story/2003/12/augusto-boals-theatre-of-the-oppressed/

Blackless, M e.a.(2000): How sexually dimorphic we are? Review and synthesis. *American Journal of Human Biology*, 12: 151–166.

Case, K., Stewart, B., & Tittsworth, J. (2009). Transgender across the curriculum: A psychology for inclusion. *The Teaching of Psychology*, 36(2): 117–121.

Cass, V. C. (1979). Homosexual identity formation: Testing a theoretical model. *Journal of Sex Research*, 1984(20): 143–167.

Castro-Peraza, M., García-Acosta, J., Delgado, N., Perdomo-Hernández, A., Sosa-Alvarez, M., Llabrés-Solé, R., & Lorenzo-Rocha, N. (2019). Gender identity: The human right of depathologization. *International Journal of Environmental Research and Public Health*, 16(6): 978. doi: 10.3390/ijerph16060978

Ciocca, G., Zauri, S., Limoncin, E., Mollaioli, D., D'Antuono, L., & Carosa, E. et al. (2020). Attachment style, sexual orientation, and biological sex in their relationships with gender role. *Sexual Medicine*, 8(1): 76–83. doi: 10.1016/j.esxm.2019.09.001

Cochran, S. D. (2001). Emerging issues in research on lesbians' and gay men's mental health: Does sexual orientation really matter? *American Psychologist*, 56: 931–947.

Coleman E. (1981–1982). The developmental stages of the coming out process. *Journal of Homosexuality*, 7(2–3): 31–43.

Coleman, E., Adler, R., Bockting, W., Botzer, M., Brown, G., Cohen-Kettenis, P., & Zucker, K. (2011). *Standards of care for the health of transgender, transgender, and gender-nonconforming people.* (7th ed.) The World Professional Association for Transgender Health. Retrieved from www.wpath.org/documents/StandardsofCareV7-2011WPATH.pdf

Corrigan, P. W., & Watson, A. C. (2002). Understanding the impact of stigma on people with mental illness. *World Psychiatry*, 1(1): 16–20.

Jacobs, L., & Hycner, R. (Eds). (2009). *Relational approaches in gestalt therapy.* New York: Gestalt Press/Routledge. Taylor & Francis Group.

Kincel, A. & Istituto di Gestalt HCC Italy (2021). Exploring masculinity, sexuality, and culture in gestalt therapy. Retrieved 6 September 2021, from www.gestaltitaly.com/exploring-masculinity-sexuality-and-culture-in-gestalt-therapy-adam-kincel/

Simington, J. A. (2019). Evaluating trauma education designed within a spiritual framework. *Journal of Humanistic Psychology*, 63(1). Retrieved from https://journals.sagepub.com/doi/10.1177

Chapter 5

Experiment and Phenomenology in Treating Gender Dysphoria

Rebecca Waletich

I am a cisgender, pansexual, white woman from the United States. This piece is informed professionally by my reading, study, and consultations with gender diverse mentors, leaders and peers, and personally by my gender diverse friends and spouse.

Gestalt therapy has components that are uniquely suited for work with the gender diverse population, including:

- a focus on organism in environment,
- attunement to our own and the client's body phenomenon, and
- the ability to use:
  - phenomenological experience,
  - relational dynamics,
  - and experiments.

This chapter will explore:

- the commonalities between the experience of trauma and the experience of gender dysphoria,
- ways Trauma-Informed Care[1] can be incorporated into the treatment of gender dysphoria,
- the importance and challenges to establishing safety, inside and outside therapy,
- the benefits and risks of phenomenological awareness in treating gender dysphoria,
- preparing the therapist for work with people with gender dysphoria,
- and ways to use gestalt theory and techniques to help clients expand awareness and heal from trauma.

Gender Dysphoria and Trauma

When the shell we stare at in the mirror does not match the person we are, when others see that shell, and make wildly wrong and hurtful assumptions, when others react to our body with rejection, pity, shame, vitriol, and

DOI: 10.4324/9781003335344-5

violence, we can feel betrayed by our own bodies. Our very body itself can become an inescapable trauma trigger.

At first blush, when people see the words gender dysphoria and trauma, I imagine they think about the gender diverse people who have experienced overt trauma. I would suggest it is more complicated than that. Over the years, my studies, and my clients, have taught me that gender dysphoria and trauma are inextricably tied. I would assert that gender dysphoria *is* a trauma. The concepts and stories detailed in this writing will start to flesh out this assertion. As you read, I invite you to experiment with interchanging the words 'gender dysphoria' with the word 'trauma' and see if that reframe changes the way you conceptualize your care.

I want to be clear that gender diversity is not trauma, dysphoria is. If there was a world, a field, in which gender diversity existed without oppression, then, it could be argued that the experience of gender dysphoria might exist without trauma, but this world is theoretical. Bias and oppression are ubiquitous. Even in this imaginary dream land, for some, dysphoria can still cause trauma. Consider the experience of a young woman I worked with, who, for a brief time, one could argue, lived in such a 'gender bias free' world.

> When I was a kid, I did not have any dysphoria. We lived out in the woods. Mom home schooled. All of my siblings and I, regardless of gender, were all just playing in the dirt, collecting bugs, climbing trees. We were all literally treated the same, until puberty hit like a freight train. My body started changing, but it was changing wrong. Imagine you were slowly growing into a cockroach. That's what it felt like. I hated my body. It disgusted me. It betrayed me, and I was powerless to stop it.

This story exemplifies one way that for those with strong body dysphoria, trauma can exist without gendered bias or oppression.

Physiological Responses to Gender Dysphoria

In support of my assertion that gender dysphoria is trauma, let's discuss some of the body responses. Gender diverse people report gender dysphoria bringing on fight/flight/freeze responses, including but not limited to, sweating, increased heart rate, hyperarousal, numbness, mental fog, and nausea (Erickson-Schroth 2014). Also, gender diverse people have a higher rate of self-harm, disordered eating, drug and/or alcohol abuse, and panic attacks than the cis population (i.e. people identifying with the gender registered at birth) (Institute of Medicine 2011).

For many gender diverse people (like many other survivors of trauma) disassociation from one's body can be a common creative adjustment. Often, disassociation is an attempt to numb the autonomic responses to outside stimuli. For gender diverse people with strong body dysphoria (dysphoria specifically triggered by one's anatomy), they do not just experience the trigger as originating from outside, but their very body itself. For many, being cued to be aware of their body starts another cycle of autonomic responses, compounding on itself. In my practice I have seen that for many clients, the cue to be aware of their breath is enough to start panic and/or bring on a dissociative episode. A common gestalt response when a client has autonomic responses in session is to explore this phenomenology. As you can imagine, sometimes, for this community, that exacerbates the issue. Often, in my experience, taking the client into hyper or hypo arousal, and creating a space where they are unable to work in session. This will be discussed more later in this writing.

To further complicate this relationship with one's body, many gender diverse people spend a great deal of time and money, as well as endure intense pain, converting and altering their bodies, in an effort to increase their comfort and safety in this world. For some, this is conforming to, or even adopting, the very misconceived gender biases that harmed them to begin with.

With the potential traumatic reaction to phenomenological body awareness, and the deeply complicated philosophical, psychological, and social dynamics surrounding their physical reality, how do we do the work of building awareness without re-traumatization or reinforcing harmful societal messages? In a word, carefully.

Trauma-Informed Care teaches us that the first step toward healing is to establish whatever level of safety is possible, both inside and outside of therapy (Taylor 2014; Yeager 2013). If, outside of the therapy room, the unsafe situation is still active in their lives, helping them reconnect to the body, might leave them vulnerable to situations that may be overwhelming for them. They may still need that creative adjustment to survive. This is true for all people experiencing trauma of any kind, but for gender diverse people, it is additionally complicated by the dynamics inherent in the threat. Let's explore some of these dynamics.

Dynamics That Complicate Safety for Gender Diverse People

The threat to gender diverse people is interwoven into society, and into our very bodies, down to a cellular level (Anodea 2004). The therapist understanding this is vital in helping create whatever level of safety is possible for the client, so it is worth taking a moment here to scratch the surface of these intricacies.

Consider this seemingly simple question and how it spirals out to impact and complicate all areas of our lives:

"Did you have a boy or a girl?"

This is, almost invariably, the first question one asks a new parent. Then, the answer to that question colors every other decision and interaction we have for, with, and about this individual. Social science is filled with articles detailing how our perception of someone's gender impacts everything from the clothes we give them, to the words we choose to use to describe the infant

("She is so pretty", "He is so strong"), to the future we encourage and support them to pursue ("She can be a great nurse", "He could be a Doctor").

Then, as we grow, these assumptions about us start to be incorporated into our understanding of ourselves, as well as our fit in the world. They have been with us so long, in overt and covert ways, that we see them as basic truths about humanity and ourselves. These biases become such a basic building block of how we order our world, and ourselves, that, for the cis population, questioning gender's link to biological sex, often feels like a personal, foundational assault to who we are. It can feel as mentally disorienting as if someone says we actually 'drop things up' and can feel as threatening as if someone is ripping the very foundation of all we are out from under us. The gender diverse person represents, by their very existence, evidence that we have built our societal and often personal foundations with faulty bricks. Humans often do not react well to this sort of truth, and take it out on the gender diverse persons and community, who are simply trying to live their own authentic truths.

As a result, a gender diverse person gets countless messages that they are wrong, their experience invalid, and that their very existence is a threat to this world. This manifests in myriad ways in every moment of their life because gendered messages are everywhere. Look around you right now. If there are people around you, do you see color differences in their attire that seem to be based on gender? Is your room decorated masculinely or femininely? What does that even mean? As ridiculous as it might seem, it is undeniable that things like a curve in the design of a chair gives people a masculine or feminine feel, based on a million tiny messages gathered from a million places. All of these messages are present in every moment. Most cis people are simultaneously immersed in, and oblivious to, this truth. Gender diverse people do not have the luxury of oblivion.

This phenomenon is just one string on the complicated knotted ball of phenomena that binds gender diverse people. Understanding the dynamic outlined above is important, because that understanding starts to draw out how and why even 'progressive' and 'enlightened' therapists are inevitably tangled into the dynamics that threaten our clients, and why we must constantly and vigilantly work to comb through our thoughts and somatic responses to help free our clients from the strings we hold. If we do not continually do our work, we will inevitably micro-aggress against our clients. (For more discussion on microaggressions from a gestalt theory perspective see "Thoughts on Microaggressions, Socio Cultural Trauma, and the Phenomenological Field", in the June 2020 edition of The New Gestalt Voices).

Detangling Ourselves

It is always important for the therapist to attend to their own bodies and somatic experience (Clemmons et al. 2008). Typically, we may think of this as important mostly for the quality of our services to our clients. For gender diverse clients, it is vital to protect against inadvertently re-traumatizing them. Through our bodies and somatic experiences, we become aware of our own internalized gendered stereotypes and biases. We, like all humans, treat people differently based on the way we have gendered people in our minds. For example, do we lean in closer to people we believe to be women? If so, how are we sitting with this woman who was assigned male at birth who may still have many of the markers that we have been taught to see as masculine? Are we subtly putting those messages in our body language, or choice of words? And in this subtle mannerism, what are we communicating to our client, who, as a result of the gendered trauma they experience, are hypersensitive of the gendered biases of which we have been blissfully oblivious?

Working with the gender diverse population provides a wonderful opportunity for the therapist to notice the subtle, but real and meaningful, ways they treat people of different gender identities differently. Then we can explore why we do this, and if that behavior serves our clients, us, or this world. This internal work not only benefits our gender diverse clients, but cis clients as well, and it can enrich our own lives.

A client, who I will call Katie (a trans woman), shared with me a subtle nonverbal that was outside of my awareness. She said,

> Pre-transition, when a group of women passed me, they would look at me for a moment, smile quickly then divert their eyes. I became aware that women did not do this with other women. They would hold eye contact, and smile warmly, even when they were strangers. It was like they were all in some exclusive club, that I was unable to be a part of. Today, a group of women passed me and smiled, like I am now a part of their club.

Her mention of this made me aware of the differences in the length of eye contact, and the way I would (or wouldn't) smile at people. She was right. For me, smiling and holding eye contact for extended periods of time with men felt vulnerable. I started being conscious of that when I worked with trans women who either were choosing to, or had to, outwardly express masculinity. I struggled to hold eye contact in the same way that I did people who outwardly expressed as feminine. Personally, this awareness betrayed some valuable work that I needed to take to my therapist. Professionally, I have learned that having been immersed in the gendered world, seeing things that are coded masculine (facial hair, certain cuts of clothes) cues my subconscious to act as if I were sitting with a man. I have learned, when I am with a gender diverse client, to notice the things that are not so steeped in gendered social conditioning (their eyes, their smile). This helps me see them, even when they are presenting in a way we have been taught to see as gendered.

Some of the ways we can help ourselves with this work is to:

- Immerse ourselves in trans culture, literature, and movies made by gender diverse people themselves. Consider following gender diverse YouTubers and bloggers. Doing this gives us opportunities to explore our own phenomenological reactions to messages, images, and ideas, before we encounter them in session.
- Seek out and reach out to community-led support groups and organizations. Ask for ways you can collaborate with and support these organizations. This work with them will not only serve the community's needs but will give you the opportunity to learn while serving.
- Join local or online professional organizations for professionals who work with gender diverse individuals. The World Professional Association for Transgender Health (WPATH), the organization that writes the Standards of Care (SOC), is an important organization to join to stay abreast of best practices in gender diverse care.[2] Psychological associations often have committees that focus on these issues. Local hospitals may have gender clinics that will collaborate with community professionals to network and share resources.
- Hire a gender diverse consultant to provide consultation on gender related issues. This is an important consideration any time we work with an oppressed population that we are not a member of. Now, with video conferencing options, we are less restricted by location, so it is easier than ever to find gender diverse people who are interested in providing this service.

Self-care

As enriching as this work is, it can also be taxing. We are stripping ourselves down to the core, examining our fundamental building blocks and deconstructing how we see the world and ourselves. This takes an emotional toll. In addition to that internal work, as with all traumatized clients, safety considerations need to be expressly and patiently cultivated. Safety looks different for every person. Cultivating an experience of safety with this population can, at times, be a journey filled with smaller steps, and more retreats, than a therapist might be accustomed to. This can leave a therapist feeling self-doubt, or unsatisfied with their own work.

To augment our usual support/selfcare plans, therapists who do this work often benefit from finding other therapists who also do work with the gender diverse community for supervision or the therapist's own therapy. This gives the therapist a sounding board to deepen their self-examination. It also helps give them support for the therapeutic and personal challenges that can come from the pacing of the sessions. Peers or supervisors who are not experienced in this area may not be able to serve this need. They often get caught in their own gendered biases, and/or are unaware of the complicated phenomena that impact treatment.

Breaking Ourselves out of the Binary

As an artifact of our brains creating a binary world often both clients and therapists are stuck in a binary understanding of gender (man/woman). I assert nothing in this world is actually as simple as our binary brains would like to believe. Very few people are brilliant, and very few are complete idiots. Very few people are at the top of the height chart, and very few are at the bottom. Most of us are spread out through the middle of life's many bell-shaped curves. People are starting to become more aware that gender also defies our binary understanding, but professionals and professional journals are lagging behind. I, and many of my peers, have found it to be important to explore our own gender identities. In this exploration, many of us, though we may identify as cis, find we are not on the extreme ends of this bell-shaped curve. It is a complicated exploration, full of many philosophical twists and quandaries, but it is worthwhile. The process itself helps us better understand some of the things our clients are trying to explain to us.

Common Triggers for Gender Dysphoria

Building safety with gender diverse clients is the first step. I draw from Taylor's work on trauma (2014) to achieve this. In addition, with the gender diverse population, I make some specific efforts, including:

- giving the client language for experiences that they may have been unable to speak about,
- normalizing these experiences,
- showing that I am aware of gender diverse peoples' struggles,
- demonstrating that I am open to discussing these topics,
- and helping the client build awareness into experiences that they were so accustomed to that they were desensitized to the discomfort they experienced (this dynamic is discussed below).

The following are some common triggers that are important for the therapist to have thought through in order to be comfortable discussing them in session as needed (see also Erickson-Schroth 2014):

- Addressing gendered ruptures: You will at some point misgender or misname a client. Pronoun and name mistakes happen. You will also accidentally, or unknowingly, endorse one of the countless gendered stereotypes you have absorbed from the environment around you. In order to honor the client's right to self-determination and affirm their status as the expert on their own needs, I recommend asking your client how they want you to repair these anticipatable ruptures before they happen. Most clients want a quick apology and immediate correction. Some may then need some sort of check-in and aftercare from the therapist. Others may ask you explicitly not to mention the rupture because the check-in can increase the discomfort. Contracting your response prior to the rupture is a useful technique to build trust and speed repair. It is a way for the client to expand awareness around how they want to coach others to respond when others misname or misgender them. I often frame this as an experiment: "Imagine I have mistakenly misgendered or misnamed you." Then exploring this with questions like "What comes up for you?", "What are you aware of?", "What does that feeling want to say to me?", "What do you need to repair this rupture?"

- Genitals and other body parts: Talking about genitals is often necessary in the therapy session. Ask after what terms the client wants you to use for genitals. Some people prefer medical terms, others will call their genitals by the term that fits their gender identity. For example, a person who was assigned female at birth, and identifies as male or non-binary, may refer to their chest, and not use the word breasts, or a female who was assigned male at birth may refer to her clitoris, and not use the word penis. There are endless other words a person may choose, so always ask.
- Sex: In addition to language about genitals, how the genitals are used can be a very difficult topic. Since sex ed is cis-hetero normative, it is important for the therapist to educate themselves and build their own internal comfort discussing this topic. Mentioning sex as a possible topic of discussion and explaining why it is important in the safety contracting phase, can help open the door to talk about this topic if it becomes figural later in the client's work. All the intricacies that can prepare a therapist to talk about sex is outside the scope of this writing. (A place to start educating yourself is referenced below: Cavanaugh 2019.)
- Religion: For many gender diverse people, their religious institutions have abused, rejected, and shamed them. As a result, discussing their experience and if, or how, the therapist might utilize any religious or spiritual tools in the work is important.
- Touch: A client once said to me, "When my body is touched, I remember 'this *is* my body', and I recoil." Some of the gender diverse people I have worked with have been so averse to touch, that even touching an object another person is also touching is overwhelming. Since some experiments may involve touch, this is an important aspect to negotiate early, and check-in on often.

Often during safety contracting, people may not endorse issues with the above, or other common gender dysphoria inducing topics. As the gender diverse person starts to allow themselves to live authentically, some experience an increased amount of dysphoria, temporarily. Imagine you have carried a shield your whole life (in this case pretending to be your gender assigned at birth). People have been throwing rocks at you for as long as you can remember (the wrong name, the wrong pronouns, the wrong expectations), but they hit the shield. The ricochet is not comfortable, but it does not hurt. With time the shield gets heavy. It slows you down. You are tired of no one seeing you behind it, so, you put it down. You may be elated to be seen, and relieved of the heavy weight of the shield, but those rocks hurt. When they called you 'he' and you were holding the 'man' shield, that was one thing, but now that they see the woman you are, hearing 'he' hits so much harder. Your awareness is no longer shielded. This increased awareness is one common reason for the temporary uptick in discomfort. Due to factors like this, safety contracting is never 'done'. The safety contracting process needs to be kept open and re-examined continually throughout treatment.

Transition as Experiment

Often clients ask, "How can I be sure I need to transition before I uproot my entire life?" They are less than pleased when I tell them no one is ever 100 percent sure of anything. Gender transition is a dance. You can watch others, think about, and plan the steps, but it takes stepping out on the floor to find your own rhythm. Maybe you work up the courage, then rush to the middle of the floor, or maybe you dance inconspicuously on the edges for a while, but whatever method you choose, it is the movement, the experiment itself, that tells you if or how you move in this dance.

Every gender diverse person's dance is their own. Each dance includes different transition steps. For some, these steps are completely internal. For others, they may not even define their movement towards authenticity as a transition at all. As a result, 'step' style developmental frameworks cannot completely capture the complexities of a human's experience. With that limitation noted, we do still reap benefits as therapists when using models of development from which to start to understand other's experiences. Arlene Istar Lev (2004), in her book *Transgender Emergence* uses a model of transition that can be useful.

1   Awareness: In this stage of awareness, people are often in great distress; the therapeutic task is the normalization of the experiences involved in emerging [gender] experience.
2   Seeking information/Reaching out: In this stage, people seek to gain education and support about [gender diversity]; the therapeutic task is to facilitate linkages and encourage outreach.
3   Disclosure to significant others: This stage involves the disclosure of their [gender identity] to significant others – spouses, partners, family members, and friends; the therapeutic task involves supporting the person's integration in the familial or community systems.
4   Exploration – Identity and Self-Labeling: This stage involves the exploration of various [gender] identities; the therapeutic task is to support the articulation and comfort with one's [gender] identity.

5 Exploration – Transition issues/possible body modification: This stage involves exploring options for transition regarding identity, presentation, and body modification; the therapeutic task is the resolution of the decisions, and advocacy towards their manifestation.
6 Integration – Acceptance and post-transition issues: In this stage the person is able to integrate and synthesize [gender] identity; the therapeutic task is support in adaptation to transition related issues.

One may notice aspects of the contact cycle (sensation, awareness, mobilization, action, contact, withdrawal/satisfaction/integration (Zinker 1977, 11)) in Lev's work. I would suggest the contact cycle is happening over and over throughout Lev's model.

I encourage you to hold these transition stages loosely in your work. There will be moments where people are in more than one stage at a time. For example, a client came to me, who I will call Abbey, reporting to be solidly in stage 5 (exploring body modifications), and seeking a vaginoplasty. Due to funding issues, Abbey's surgery was delayed for a year. Over that year, she affirmed how intensely she wanted this surgery both in words and actions. Abbey changed jobs to be able to afford it, moved and got a roommate to save money. She also quit smoking and lost 50 pounds all to prepare for surgery. She was determined! I remember the day the funding finally came through. I handed her the letter she needed from me for her insurance to cover the procedure. She welled up with tears like I was handing her a golden ticket. Then, a week later, in her next session, smiling, clear-eyed and looking lighter and less burdened than I had ever seen her before, she said,

> My entire adult life, surgery was my goal. It was the 'final step'. Everyone told me, and I believed, that all women have vaginas, so I was not a woman. Then, the moment your letter touched my hand I knew, like it was always there just beneath the fog. I am happy with my body. My penis is useful. I enjoy it. I am a chick with a dick!
> (Retelling that story, I get chills, and happy tears, like I did the day she said it.)

Her story illustrates how people can be in many of Lev's stages of transition at a time. Abbey was growing awareness of her gender experience (stage 1) through exploration of body modifications (stage 5) leading to integration (stage 6). If the therapist tries to put the client in these stages in a rigid or linear way, the therapist is making contact with the model, not the client.

If held loosely though, these stages can help therapists understand some of the experiences of their clients. Then, together, the therapist and client can co-create safe experiments, for both in and outside of session. Below we will discuss examples of experiments.

Examples of Experiments: Providing and Advocating for Affirming Care

The second thing that Abbey's story illustrates is the importance of affirming care. Abbey shared with me that prior to having the ability to get her surgery all she could think about was how to make it happen. She was so busy connecting with the barriers to her surgery that she was unable to be aware of anything else. I hear one of my gestalt instructors, Steve Roberts, LCSW, in my head. He would always remind us that organisms know how to heal, and that our job is simply to help them clear a way through their introjects to become aware of what they already know. By believing what she said, that she needed surgery, and helping her clear away the obstacles to surgery, she was able to see what was always there "beneath the fog" as she said. When I teach live classes, and tell Abbey's story, many therapists get hung up on if her story means we should slow the process down, and do more to *make sure* the client is 'sure'. I think it illustrates the opposite. The barriers blocked her awareness. If the therapist becomes a barrier (or as the community says a 'gate keeper'), they are working against their client. Affirming care, and advocating for your client, is not just the best practices according to the WPATH SOC, it is an opportunity for the client to expand awareness of self.

Verbalizing Attunement

Verbalizing the therapist's attunement can be a useful skill to prepare the client for future awareness work. In the early stages, this needs to be done gently and cautiously. The experience of being seen is often scary for gender diverse people. This is not unusual for survivors of trauma. Specifically, for gender diverse people, it can trigger gender-based fears about 'what' you (the therapist) see, and how you have gendered them. You will find that a high percentage of gender diverse clients choose to spend much of their social capital in online worlds. Sometimes it may be virtual online worlds like The Sims, and Second Life. Other times they have most of their contact in the form of social media platforms. This allows them to create the persona that fits their inner reality, as well as creates the safety derived from anonymity. As a result, in-person contact can be incredibly intense. Gender diverse people often express longing to be seen, and touched, but find it overwhelming and frightening. This is yet another experience that survivors of all sorts of trauma can relate to. The simple act of noticing a twitch on their face can trigger a cascade of feelings, and autonomic reactions, that the client is unable to regulate in the moment.

Body Awareness

The body is a reservoir full of information gathered from experience, environment, and biology. As discussed earlier, for clients who experience gender dysphoria, especially ones with strong body dysphoria, disassociation from one's body is a common creative adjustment. By disconnecting from one's body, they may reduce the immediate experience of suffering, but they deny themselves needed information to help them establish and live an authentic life. Experiment is an important tool to help the client access this phenomenological somatic information and power. In my work, I start with first teaching clients why this is important. This teaching is important for buy in. Clients have reported that without this explanation, the invitation to be aware of their body 'just seems cruel'. Then we slowly co-create experiments. For example, with one client, we began by them touching different textured cloth with the tips of their fingers, asking them to feel the cloth, and be aware of the sensation, just in their fingers, while staying present to the moment and their breath. This 'simple' experiment took weeks to do before they were able to stay present and notice their fingers without strong dissociation. For inspiration, even with adults, I draw from children's resources, like *Windows to Our Children* (Oaklander 1989) on ways to grade experiments way down.

Language

It is important to use pronouns, gendered language, and chosen names in session, as well as to find or create spaces for them to be used outside of session. This activity provides opportunity to explore the somatic experience of hearing these words. Even if the client is unsure about the exact pronouns or name that they would like used at that moment, explore ways to use the gendered words, trying them on if you will, to see how they feel. A way to grade this experiment down might be avoiding pronouns completely or using neutral pronouns like 'they/them/theirs' or 'zi/zim/zeirs'. It is possible to use pronouns even when talking to the person. For example, rewording sentences like instead of saying "I wonder if you would ...", say "I was thinking 'I wonder if she would ....'"

Art

This is an area with countless possibilities. Some examples of artistic experiments include inviting the client to:

- Create a visual or imagined image of the gender role they were assigned at birth. Is it a shell, a shield, a trap, a costume etc.? Explore what comes up when looking at that creation from the outside. What is it like to exist in this shell?
- Create collages to start to visualize what the client wants to be included in their authentic expression, like a 'vision board'.
- Use artistic medium (paint, clay, fabric, really anything) to make tangible the felt experience of living authentically. Use experiment to interact with these artistic creations, to understand, and integrate the experience that inspired it.

- Collect pictures of self over lifetime. "Do you see yourself in them?", "What was the experience like for the person in the picture?", "If you could tell them something, what would you want them to know?" etc.
- Create a visual 'field of dysphoria'. Have them write, or draw, dysphoria triggers, or gender related introjects on separate slips of paper. Then place them around the room in a way that makes sense for them (maybe placing them farther if they want them farther, or closer if they feel more intense). With this, one could go many directions, including: sitting with awareness of this visual representation of the field, talking to the manifestations of their introjects, or moving them to where they would rather these introjects be. This experiment is one that I do repeatedly through my work with people. It is useful to process what has left the field or become more important with evolving awareness.

Gender Expression

The therapy room can be used as a safe space for external gender expression (clothing, mannerisms, etc.). A client may change in the restroom prior to session, or dress in layers before they come into the office. They may apply make-up, put their hair into a hat, or otherwise alter their look in session as the therapist uses phenomenological tools to build somatic awareness. I encourage therapists to have mirrors available. Mirrors should not be situated in a way that the client is unable to avoid seeing themselves. Seeing a reflection can be very upsetting to some clients, so they need to be able to actively consent to seeing their reflection.

Roleplay and Two Chair Work

In the office, the client can roleplay 'coming out' conversations, standing up for oneself, or other difficult situations. Together you can negotiate how the therapist might join in the role play. Perhaps as an advocate, an unaccepting voice, or maybe therapist as client themselves.

Two chair work can be a powerful experimental modality. This could be designed to work on the polarity between:

- the part of them that is scared to come out and the part that is eager to live authentically;,
- the 'old them' and the 'new them';
- what gender is to them verses what society says gender is;
- or the 'feminine' and 'masculine'.

A common time when I find two chair to be useful is when a client is stuck in 'what ifs' (what if I regret this later, what if I have a medical complication, etc.). I ask them to imagine the later them, who is not happy with present them and invite them to put that person in the other chair. As a variation of this, I often invite them to physically write a letter to this future self, explaining why they made the choice they are currently making. This process allows them to look at the present decision in a different manner, to either cement it, or reconsider it. It also can alleviate some anxiety to have this physical letter to know they can remind themselves later that they made the best decision they could at the time with what they knew.

In my practice, I often delay inviting two chair work on the polarity between the binary genders (masculine and feminine) until a later stage of work, in the Acceptance and Integration stage. Early on there is often a visceral pushing away of the birth gender, and the suggestion of acknowledging the parts of them that align with the birth gender can be misread as the therapist trying to make them accept that they are this gender. In the Acceptance and Integrations stages, gender diverse people often are working to integrate the parts of them that align with the gender assigned at birth with their life post transition (i.e. "can I, as a woman, still like working on cars?"), so inviting work on the feminine and masculine can be useful. Two chair work between the masculine and the feminine can also be very useful with nonbinary clients as a tool to negotiate their authentic experience outside the binary, with the world they exist in that has taught them to gender things inside of themselves in a binary way.

Breaking the Binary

As discussed earlier, many times people are stuck in a binary idea of gender. This can create challenges. Let's oversimplify gender for a moment. Imagine gender was on a 1–10 continuum, 1 = woman, 10 = man. If a client is stuck in the artificial constrains of a gender binary, they may know "I am not a woman" and then assume "I must be a man." So they may, with this understanding, run as fast as they can from 1 to 10. But let's imagine this person's gender identity is actually a 7.5. This 'overcorrection' (going to 10) can be confusing and frustrating. I have found that introducing the idea of identities outside of the binary and inviting people to imagine transition as a journey that can speed, slow, turn, or stop can be useful. It does not necessarily stop people from making steps they later decide to walk back on. It shouldn't stop that. That process is part of learning. What it does seem to do, is lessen their discomfort when turns on the road do need to be made, so they can find the path that is their own a slight bit easier.

Gender Euphoria

Gender euphoria refers to the joy, excitement, and/or satisfaction that one gets when they are able to live in their authentic truth. I find often that my clients are so conditioned to see their gender as an 'issue' or a 'problem' that they are shocked to hear this experience exists. Introducing this idea and bringing it into therapy can be useful. The invitation to imagine this experience can be powerful. Sometimes I find it helps clients identify and expand this feeling outside of session, other times it brings out deep despondence and disbelief that they will ever have this experience.

In Conclusion

This professional journey, for all its difficult internal untangling, slow and arduous safety work, and painful truths, has led me to some of the most fulfilling experiences in my life. Let me conclude with a client story, in her own words. My hope is that you will see in her words the value of what gestalt practice has to offer this population in connecting with their bodies and experiences:

> Before I came out, I saw people as attractive, but the idea of being touched made me recoil, so much so that I believed I just didn't like to be touched. It didn't really make sense though, because as a very young child I was a cuddler. I always wanted to be in someone's lap or hugged. After I came out and started to find things I liked about my body, I started to yearn to be touched. I realized that before, when I was touched, it was a tactile reminder of what I was not happy with about my body. Now, I am learning how to engage intimately with people all over again, or really for the first time, as me. Things that sound like they would be so simple, like hugging a friend goodbye, or cuddling up watching a movie with a date, seemed hard somehow, like I am teaching my limbs a foreign language, one that I ached to speak.

About Rebecca Waletich

Rebecca Waletich, LCSW (she/her) has been serving LGBTQIA adults and youth since 1999. Rebecca is the owner and a therapist at Transformations Counseling Services, a group practice that provides individual, couples, family, and group therapy for Gender Diverse youth and adults. Rebecca is a WPATH Certified Therapist and Mentor. Outside of her practice, she is active in advocacy, professional training, and networking efforts. Rebecca facilitates a clinical consultation group, Queer Clinical Consultation for therapists who need support in their work with Gender Diverse clients. Rebecca collaborates with Riley Hospital Gender Clinic and the BU Wellness Network as a case consultant to their gender service programs. Rebecca is an active member of the National Association of Social Workers Sexual Orientation and Gender Identity Committee. Rebecca is a member of AAGT, has completed three years of gestalt training at the Indiana Gestalt Institute, and has trained with GALTA in Seattle.

Notes

1 Trauma-Informed Care (TIC) is an approach in the human service field that assumes that an individual is more likely than not to have a history of trauma. Trauma-Informed Care recognizes the presence of trauma symptoms and acknowledges the role trauma may play in an individual's life – including service staff.
2 WPATH, like all large organizations, is not without controversy. Despite that, the evidence based, affirming, client centered care that they advocate is accepted as best practices by many global medical associations, and all major US insurance companies. As such, it is important to be aware of the WPATH SOC.

References

Anodea, Judith. *Eastern Body, Western eMind: Psychology and the Chakra System as a Path to the Self/ Potter*/Ten Speed/Harmony/Rodale; Revised ed. Edition August 1, 2004.

Cavanaugh, T. "Sexual Health History: Talking Sex with Gender Non-Conforming & Trans Patients". *Fenway Health* 2019. https://fenwayhealth.org/wp-content/uploads/Taking-a-Sexual-Health-History-Cavanaugh-1.pdf. Date of Access 1/26/2020

Clemmons, M., Frank, R., & Smith, E. "Somatic Experience and Emergent Dysfunction: Gestalt Therapists in Dialogue from the Editors and with Eugene Gendlin." *Studies in Gestalt Therapy*, vol. 2, no. 2, 2008, pp. 11–39.

Erickson-Schroth, L. (Ed.). *Trans Bodies, Trans Selves: A Resource for the Transgender Community*. Oxford University Press. 2014.

Institute of Medicine (US). Committee on Lesbian, Gay, Bisexual, and Transgender Health Issues and Research Gaps and Opportunities. *The Health of Lesbian, Gay, Bisexual, and Transgender People: Building a Foundation for Better Understanding*. National Academies Press (US). 2011. Available from: www.ncbi.nlm.nih.gov/books/NBK64806/ doi: 10.17226/13128

Lev, Arlene. *Transgender Emergence: Therapeutic Guidelines for Working with Gender-Variant People and Their Families*. The Haworth Clinical Practice Press. 2004.

Oaklander, Violet. *Windows to Our Children: Gestalt Therapy Approach to Children and Adolescents*. Gestalt Journal Press. 1989.

Taylor, Miriam. *Trauma Therapy and Clinical Practice: Neuroscience, Gestalt and the Body*. McGraw Hill Education, Open University Press. 2014.

Yeager, K. R. *Modern Community Mental Health an Interdisciplinary Approach*. Routledge. 2013.

Zinker, Joseph. *Creative Process in Gestalt Therapy*. Brunner/Mazel Publishers. 1977.

Chapter 6

'Selfish and Destructive'

Where Does the Late-in-Life Lesbian Seek Therapeutic Support?

Miriam Grace

> I had [a therapist] that said being gay was 'no big deal' to her. She was trying to comfort me that she wouldn't be judgemental but when you've dealt with homophobia you also want it to be a big deal to your therapist. I was trying to talk about how it wrecked my life and I felt she was dismissive.

There is an increase in the number of women coming out later in life. Growing up in a homophobic and sexist society has created a tendency in women, currently in midlife, to consider others' needs before their own, to take a larger part of the physical, domestic and emotional load in creating families and homes, and in not viewing herself as a sexual person. These potential clients are grappling with ageism, sexism and homophobia not just of the 2020s but of the post-war idealism their culture was steeped in half a century ago. Female suppressed, emerging or fluid, sexuality is likely to have been seen as a threat to the fabric of society.

Therapy is an opportunity whereby people have a chance to experience developmental processes, such as exploration of their sexuality, that they were unable to access at key stages in their lives. Often invisible and masked by more obvious issues, a middle-aged woman's sexuality may not be on a therapist's radar given the context of the therapist's own prejudice and bias and that of psychotherapy training.

Deciding to consider herself (within the context of her own and others' expectations) is 'self-ish' and this may result in a realisation of her sexuality and/or the de-structuring of a carefully composed 'nuclear family' unit. Her therapist may be called upon to support a 'self-ish' exploration that leads to the dismantling of the structures around her (mobilising 'destruction').

This chapter is a summary of ethnographic research among later-in-life lesbian women and their therapy. (For the sake of this chapter, 'later-in-life lesbian' is a cis straight woman over 40 who discovers unexpectedly, or decides finally, that she is now lesbian.) It concludes with thoughts as to why creative gestalt therapy is well placed to offer good therapy to this client group.

I am grateful for the generous sharing of stories within an anonymous group of over 2,000 later-in-life lesbians and also through discussions with

DOI: 10.4324/9781003335344-6

Andrea Hewitt, Alison Lake and Anne-Marie Zanzal, all of whom have published material about supporting women coming out as lesbian in later life. Anonymous quotes from later-in-life lesbians are included. Opinions and conclusions are mine and are not intended to represent a group opinion.

Who Is the 'Later-in-Life Lesbian'?

A common assumption is that the later-in-life lesbian has been closeted and has finally found the courage to come out, 'better late than never'. While this is true of a few participants in this study, it was by no means a majority. While some had always known they were lesbian and a change in society or a change in their personal circumstances (such as death of a parent or children leaving home) enabled them to come out, far more women reported a fluidity (see also Diamond, 2012) and a distinct change in their sexual attraction. These women often experienced being taken by surprise when they fell in love with a woman and may initially have believed this to be a 'one off', before coming to the conclusion that their sexuality itself had changed. A third, but not final, category is that many can now see that they were lesbian before this but did not understand or conceptualise it as such. It is not uncommon for women who have married a man and had a family, to fall in love with a woman and form a new relationship (see also Diamond, 2012).

> For me the problem was not to find a LGTB friendly therapist but to find one who understood the 'coming out late in life' process.

Realising Later in Life: "How Did You Not Know?"

This question can indicate criticism, usually unintentional, that implies the lesbian was irresponsible or stupid to not know. Family, partners and friends may express hurt or anger that the woman did not share her emerging insights or confusion along the way, as if the new lesbian has been deceitful rather than evolving a very personal and private aspect of herself. The woman in question does not need to justify her sexuality or her timing to others.

Role Models and Life in the 1950s–1980s

How many of the women born in the 1950s–1980s had known of adult lesbians when they were children? How many of these women had known in teenage years or when they married a man that they could have babies with or a relationship with a woman? Again and again the responses came and not one of those who responded, grew up with this known in their lives.

With religious input, inequality in women's pay and daily sexism to grind down their natural teenage passion for life, these women were also influenced by the AIDS crisis of the 1980s, which led to increased homophobia in society. Girls were taught that the safest option was to have the narrowest sexual experience possible, only one sexual partner for life, to prevent an untimely death.

The rise of popular psychology and humanistic psychology in the 1960s only added to her problems. In the hetero-normative family, it was the woman, who was expected to notice and mend any emotional problems in her spouse or children. Tasked with improving her emotionally and sexually unsatisfying relationships often resulted in her belief that lack of satisfaction was normal or due to her own failing. Unsatisfying sex might be assumed to be normal or due to religious guilt.

Women seeking a new partner in 2020, have more options, role models, permissions and life experience than they did as young adults. Making choices in midlife, the qualities, characteristics and gender of their partner may be radically different to those of 20 or 30 years ago.

> Born 1974. I didn't know any lesbians ever. I didn't even know what the term lesbian meant. I was raised growing up that you married a man and had children. The only role model I knew was *Ellen* on TV in the 80s. I will not forget when she said, "I'm gay" on the microphone on her episode.

> I was born in the 70s. I had no idea women could be gay. At 19 I came across an 'out' lesbian singer and just thought, "wow, I wish I could be like her!" But I knew I wanted a family so therefore I knew I couldn't be.

Exploring Identity

Anne-Marie Zanzal reported that a majority of new lesbians in the support groups she runs are 'femme'. Femme lesbians can often 'pass' as heterosexual in a way that 'butch' lesbians don't. This might account for butches coming out earlier as their presentation is more obvious to themselves and to others.

In addition, she and Rachel Galliard Smook observe that many of the women they support came from chaotic and disordered families and were therefore more driven to create an ordered, 'normal' family, thus skipping over the window of opportunity for authentic evolution of their identity.

Many women experience a loss of role as their children grow up and leave home. Those overly invested in their children will experience 'empty nest syndrome' (Myers & Raup, 1989) acutely as the incomplete gestalt of identity presents once more. Zanzal (2019) describes falling in love with her children as a contributory factor to her delay in learning she was lesbian. (The first 'test tube babies' were born in the 1980s, making it unheard of to have babies without a husband. Gay people were not allowed to adopt.)

Hormones

Sexual fluidity is a reality for many women. Diamond (2012) explains that the necessity within the LGBTQIA community to promote the idea that people are "born that way" is a historical way of aligning homophobia with oppression such as racism. There are many moral and legal reasons to not discriminate against LGBTQIA individuals other than whether their sexuality is chosen or predetermined. Diamond argues there is much to indicate that not all lesbians *are* born that way. One interesting observation in the later-in-life community is that the "switching teams" experience often coincides with a drop in oestrogen.

> My first therapist believed I must have repressed my sexuality somehow, but that truly wasn't the case. And when I told them that I felt like my sexuality had shifted as opposed to me uncovering something I'd repressed, they were quite sceptical.

No one is suggesting that oestrogen makes women straight, but a majority of menopausal women concur that they have decreased capacity to accept other people's standards or ideas about how they should live their lives. It is possible that a drop in oestrogen is a contributory factor for some women to be less conforming and more self-directing. The oestrogen drop can facilitate a drop of tolerance for being a second class citizen. If she associates her male partner with her loss of self she may not seek solace with him.

Motherhood is an oxytocin-laden experience with many falling in love with their babies. When the children grow up and leave home, the mother may feel her relationship with her partner is not providing bonding hormones of oxytocin. She may seek marriage counselling, she may feel lonely and lost, or she may even seek out those excellent providers of oxytocin, other women (women are often more practised at soothing tones of voice, coupled with gentle touch and empathic eye contact. Lesbianism is sometimes considered to be quite compelling due to its capacity for this mutual oxytocin-inducing behaviour).

In conclusion, the invisibility of same sex attraction in her culture growing up, often combined with devotion to motherhood, and believing her own sexuality is irrelevant, non-existent or dirty may leave a woman quite unaware of her sexuality till the space to consider herself arrives in later life. In addition, growing up too quickly (adapted child, see Berne, 1964), might add to the propensity for a younger woman skipping her adolescent exploration of her sexuality altogether. The role of hormones is not understood, but it is interesting that peri-menopause and menopause often result in changes in a woman's temperament, and it does seem this can often be a time when a woman asserts herself and that for some this self-volition seems to include coming out as lesbian. She may have a delayed exploration of her sexuality or a complete change of sexuality and quite often a combination of the two.

It is impossible to ascertain in what way the later-in-life lesbian's timing is influenced by the sexism and homophobia in society, in the society they were raised in and internalised within the lesbian herself. If society were different, would her timing be different? Would she have been lesbian all along or would she naturally have been fluid?

The question of why she came out later is for her own personal under-standing. What is more important is *how* being a lesbian affects a woman coming out later in life.

The Need for Therapy

This group of women is less in the public eye, the challenges are quite unique, the need for therapy is frequent, and little is known about this increasing phenomenon, even by the women themselves. Therapists can learn from the participants in this study in order to improve their work.

Lake's 2018 study explored the hypothesis that women who come out later-in-life experience higher rates of depression and anxiety when compared to heterosexual women:

> Once a later life lesbian was out they had the same stressors as life-long lesbians and so the chances of ongoing suffering were similar ... The costs for later life lesbians can be huge, especially those who are in het-erosexual marriages. Coming out may lead to estrangement or divorce, family breakdown, loss of custody of children, financial implications and social avoidance. The less family support a person had was positively associated with poor mental health.

The challenges faced are multiple, major stressors: divorce; estrangement from family; loss of children; empty nest syndrome; shifting identity; rela-tionship breakups; financial hardship; new relationships; house moves; attempts to re-establish a career path or financial independence; ageing and health issues; menopause; invisibility; sexism; ageism and homophobia. These issues require support.

Support Systems

The reactions of others when women who are expected to be grey and invis-ible become 'rainbow' are not always filled with joy and welcome. Closest friends might be suspicious, feeling that the new lesbian is secretive or with-holding. The community they may have turned to for support for decades, church, family, friends, work, may no longer be available yet the LGBTQIA community may also feel inaccessible.

Many new lesbians report feeling ostracised by the straight community but too afraid to try and fit into the gay community. They fear being accused of experimentation and using their straight privilege or only coming out after their lesbian sisters have fought the battle for rights and space. They feel guilty if coming out is easy and distressed if it is difficult.

Many participants lose a male partner they consider to be 'their best friend'. Parenting and stressors in their hetero life continue but support may be missing. In limbo between two worlds and belonging to neither, the resil-ience of these women is to be wondered at.

Bonding and Bond Breaking

The deepest bonds are changing, maybe with friends, husband, children and pets.

New lesbians who have spent a decade or two with a man may be prone to falling into hetero-normative roles with their new woman, finding it is hard to give up a life time of conditioning. Potential to invent new ways of living unique to the couple, without sexist power dynamics, is wonderful, but it's an easy assumption to believe this eradicates sexism.

Women reported that they wished their therapists understood how intense their affairs with women were, how beautiful, how painful and how devastating. Attachment issues re-emerge and may be surprising in their capacity to regress a mature woman's psychological responses to less resolved stances. Therapists may misunderstand the level of distress to indicate attachment disorder, without information that it is a different type of attachment and bond breaking that is new, and may feel alarming, to a client.

There is still a degree of lesbo-phobia in the way we consider certain types of bonding as normal or pathological. Lesbian attachment measured against heterosexual or male gay relationships can be judged as 'too intense'. Many women have a tremendous capacity for emotional connection and range. The echoes of 'hysteria' and the sinister undertones of committal of women for being emotional or displaying strong attachments to other women, are bound into the history of diagnosis of mental illness. Maybe lesbian relationships indicate these women's emotional maturity, capacity and strength. It's easier for therapists to diagnose attachment disorder and co-dependency than to critically evaluate the sexism and lesbo-phobia central to our concepts of normal, healthy, adult attachment.

Of course, not all women are highly expressive or emotional, and the full spectrum of lesbian behaviour and expression is evidenced. The more self-contained, undemonstrative lesbian is less likely to be categorised as hysterical, but as we have already explored, she may experience pressure to explain herself and be regarded as secretive or aloof instead.

> I have a therapist … She is fantastic with the divorce, … helping me to survive a breakup, my burgeoning sexuality, my parenting and kid issues, but she doesn't understand the intensity of lesbian relationships, the wearing down and frustration and 'otherness' that sets in when you live among primarily straight people … she doesn't understand that lesbian breakups are different.

Identity

The roles of mother and wife are clearly defined and absorbed even at pre-verbal stages and throughout life. Many later-in-life lesbians have spent a decade or more doing the school run, being known as 'Mrs', maintaining the routines of a family home. Women have not absorbed alternative role models, thus outgrowing wife and mother roles, they have to fashion their own identity without a template. The invisibility of mid-life women lends itself to radical reinvention of self, however it also points to a soul destroying reflection that she does not or cannot exist in real life as she does not exist in fiction. The role of TV programmes such as *Orange Is the New Black* or *Last Tango in Halifax* from the BBC, in helping women visualise new identities and same-gendered partners is not to be understated. Working with fixed gestalts has to involve a leap of imagination and play, an environment that doesn't demand introjection.

Someone whose development was put on hold to serve the needs of others may struggle with their identity as something individualistic. While the later-in-life lesbian may not have to deal with the danger and invisibility of her 'sisters' who came out decades ago, she may not feel 'privileged', she may feel she has been robbed of herself. Women straight or otherwise, are oppressed to a lesser or greater extent, many have had their physical safety endangered in order to access straight privilege, their bodies may have felt invaded, owned, criticised and designed by others, their intellect may have been dismissed, their confidence eroded. New lesbians can feel a huge amount of grief of having missed out on years of being their authentic self, coupled with the grief of losing the structure and privileges of straight life.

Late bloomers have a degree of internalised homophobia and sexism. In the initial stages especially, many do not want to be, or identify as, lesbian. They may dislike their authentic self. Additionally, there is often a large degree of guilt and self-blame for the impact of her sexuality on her family.

Exploring and accepting conflicting polarities as is common in gestalt helps the client to live within the place she is, limbo, and to be accepted without introjecting. Shame and disgust can be welcomed and given voice.

Middle-aged women usually emerge from divorce financially worse off than their ex-husbands. The later-in-life lesbian has often lost her financial security and may feel too old and too under-resourced to rebuild. They may find it difficult to rebuild their financial independence having relinquished important career steps to raise a family and support her husband's career.

Coming out later in life is not easier than coming out when younger, it is different. Her process of transition bears resemblance to the coming out process but is also uniquely different. Unlike the sense of being constantly 'othered' that younger lesbians may have experienced, (which with Cass [1979] would precipitate 'Identity Confusion') the later-in-life lesbian has often fitted in well. She is in limbo between the culture, community and life she has been living in and a new life that is uncertain and unknown. Comparing who has it worse is like trying to compare going blind as the result of an accident in adult life, to having been born blind.

Accessing Therapy

Therapy is not always seen as the best place to get support in the later-in-life community and I will be exploring why and considering how this could be addressed by gestalt therapists for whom creative exploration is a trademark.

Equal Treatment Is Not Equal Access: Finding Safe LGBTQIA-Friendly Therapists

It's been very difficult to access queer-friendly counsellors. I've had a counsellor tell me I can't be bisexual and dictate my sexual orientation to me.

Finding a safe therapist is a key issue when you are in a minority group, to try and avoid re-traumatisation. There were some homophobic interventions recorded, but they were rare. Unfortunately, therapists are leaving it up to clients to try and work out if the therapist is homophobic or not.

My first therapist was unhelpful – she advised me not to seek a relationship with a woman because life would get messy

Equal access takes account of the context and makes it *easier* for the oppressed group. Thus specialist training and displayed on websites or therapy profile shows which therapists are taking extra steps. Again and again these clients are saying they don't want to be treated the same because they are not the same, they have different, important and big issues.

Therapist Investment in the Client's Sexual Identity Expression

Denying sexuality, telling a person their sexuality is wrong, is an obvious oppression. Asking them if they are sure is unnecessary and can feel non-accepting. Pushing a client to celebrate and affirm their coming out before the client is ready, might seem affirming but is also harmful. Therapists must never take on defining a person's sexuality, even if the client's wavering, internalised homophobia or self-doubt is difficult to witness. The client does not need to have a label or to stick to their label. They can stay in the closet or come out and go back in again and this is hard for a therapist who is certain about their own sexuality. However, it is disempowering to pre-empt this and therapists must be wary of over-identifying or encouraging clients to come out the way they themselves did.

My therapist was invested in saving my hetero marriage because I'm a therapist and she thought I'd send more referrals, if she saved the marriage. Yuck.

The space to explore concerns stemming from the client's straight life and from her gay life is not usually available. This was the pull of online support groups for this demographic, a space where they were able to have issues from both worlds.

Minimising the Importance of Sexuality

It's also important to realise that not exploring sexuality is an issue that affects the client. Simply affirming that their sexuality is OK with you misses the point that it might not be OK with them or other people and that it impacts their life. Don't say, "That's OK, I'm supportive of gay people." Ask, "How do you think this affects you?" This shows support but more importantly, awareness of impact.

Interpreting 'Late' as Confused

It is not acceptable for a therapist to not know about the existence of later-in-life lesbians. Late does not mean that your client has got it wrong in terms of timing or attraction; her timing will make sense once her story is heard. She is allowed to be fluid or lesbian and she is allowed to do that at any time. It is not a failing or a flaw to be gay and it is not a failing to be later in life.

> Did I really just sit with a couples therapist for two and a half hours and try to convince him and my husband that I'm never having sex with a man again? No, I'm not bi; I'm not fluid; I'm not changing my mind. I'm GAY, gay, gay. It seriously felt like conversion therapy. And every time I have this discussion with every therapist (this is our third), I feel like I'm re-injuring my husband all over again. When do people finally take you at your word that you are gay?

Applying Male 'Norms' or Straight 'Norms' to Lesbian Relationships

Increased awareness that psychotherapeutic history and relationship norms are straight norms is very important and continued monitoring of oneself but also one's supervisor for archaic beliefs is important. An understanding that the intensity of lesbian relationships and breakups is not pathological would be appreciated by many of the women who spoke to me.

Judging relationship norms by straight norms is unhelpful. Ask how your client feels, ask her the pros and cons, pick up her tendency to be judgemental because it is not what she knows.

> She was just not willing to address my sexual orientation and what I was experiencing. Her take was just to be available to all. I was never sure what that was supposed to mean and I finally went looking for someone else.

Applying LGBTQIA Norms to the Client

Gay therapists are sometimes sought when the issue is clearly related to coming out, in the hope that they will understand the coming-out process.

> I truly don't know if there are straight therapists who really "get" the coming out process – not on that deep level.

But they can be overly invested in the client process.

> My gay psychologist wanted me to drop everything and move out asap.
> … a counsellor needs to leave space for a client to explore their doubts. The counsellor that I saw for about 6 months when I was in the first part of my process treated it very quickly like a forgone conclusion that I was gay, but I wasn't quite there yet. I still needed to ask the questions of myself and come to an answer. I felt like she expected a confidence in my sexuality that I just didn't have yet.

There is a need for therapeutic input and support but there is some suspicion of therapists. The therapists who most misunderstand their later-in-life lesbian clients are usually straight therapists, though a lesbian or gay therapist may have negative personal experiences of people who have lived for decades with straight privilege suddenly 'deciding to' explore their sexuality in a more permissive society than the therapist may have had to battle through in their own coming out process.

Why Gestalt?

What emerged universally was that these women's sexuality is 'a big deal' and needs to be taken seriously; that the coming out process is not a one off, completed process, but a lifelong process that colours every day; and that while straight therapists are more prone to prejudiced response, therapists who considered themselves either allies or LGBTQIA themselves can also push their views onto these clients. Gestalt is a creative therapy about fluidity, flow, exploration and client experimentation. It is well suited to work with a client who is rejecting an introjected identity and exploring options for a new identity.

Classic gestalt works with polarities, sitting with contradiction and uncomfortable feelings. It is designed to sit with uncomfortable feelings and to dialogue with different choices and options. It takes as a central premise the need for a client to describe and define themselves in their own words.

Dialogic gestalt is crucial so that the experience can be verbalised and the client can feel engaged with and not as if they are invisible or speaking into a void.

Therapy can be extremely helpful for these women as long as the therapist and supervisor are explicitly examining their bias and expectations.

I suggest that all gestalt therapists, whatever their sexual orientation, spend some creative supervision time in the lesbian chair, and find out what of the experience fits and what does not. What would it be like for the straight therapist to go home and tell everyone they are gay? And at work? How would they view their past and their marriage? What would it be like in practice, who would they need to tell? If the therapist is gay can they extend their understanding to how it might be to have not come out earlier, but to have built a straight life and to come out later? Or to those who knew they never could live a straight life, maybe they could explore how it would be now if it dawned upon them that they might be straight? How would this affect their lives?

In therapy there are many options to explore. To creatively build and dismantle a structure, feeling into the senses, exploring the imagery, connecting with taking a creation apart could be powerful. Using imagery to explore transformation and transition can be a helpful practise ground or dry run for a client embarking on change. Old therapeutic friends such as two chair work as an aid to explore internalised homophobia encourage the client to focus on their relationship with themselves. For a deepening, maturing person old style gestalt has a lot to offer someone who is freeing herself from the constraints of approval. Internal dialogue with herself and her dreams is another way that the therapist can encourage the most inexpressible of ideas into acceptance.

A humanistic therapy that explores the role of introjects in one's life, undoing retroflection and exploration as an antidote to fixed gestalts is ideally placed to support self-directed evolution towards increased personal satisfaction. The field and context is crucial and the therapist does well to be aware of their personal impact as well as that of the societal field. Inquiry and experimentation are particularly well suited to transitional process when we desire the client to find their personal truth, not our political stance.

Conclusion

If her context has not been conducive to the client being interested in her sexuality in her life so far, the potential for therapy to redress that is hopeful. The opportunity to not repeat this cultural blind spot for the client is there.

Straight and gay therapists (supervisors and trainers) have investment in their sexual identity, and can aid the process by not providing new introjects from archaic assumptions threaded through the history of psychotherapy and the society it evolved within or from current LGBTQIA politics.

If a client is a later-in-life lesbian, verbalising her truth and self-actualising, will be self-ish in that she begins to think of herself, the outcome (though she may not realise it) may involve the dismantling of her hetero-normative family structure. It is a radical act of self-regulation that will affect others and it's understandable that in weighing up the consequences many choose not to come out, or take many years looking for a compromise only to realise they cannot do otherwise. To rock the boat as a woman does when she comes out later in life, is a courageous and anti-social action. To define herself is a radical act greatly suited to gestalt.

About Miriam Grace

Miriam Grace is a gestalt psychotherapist and has been in practice for 30 years. Her enthusiasm, care and knowledge in her work with a diverse client group has facilitated her development as a practitioner integrating psychotherapy, bodywork and spirituality into her approach, seeing these all as complementary ways of engaging with being fully human.

Miriam's current research and writing is focussed on her interest in the experiences of mid-life transitions from a woman-centred perspective. Her specialist therapy groups about lesbian heart-break, menopause and coming out later in life have arisen from the lack of appropriate therapeutic support that she has come across for herself and for clients experiencing these transitions.

She is grateful for the generous sharing of stories within an anonymous group of over 2,000 later-in-life lesbians and for discussions with other authors who have published material about coming out in later life.

References

Berne, Eric (1964). *Games People Play: The Basic Hand Book of Transactional Analysis*. New York: Ballantine Books.

Cass, V. (1979). Homosexual identity formation: A theoretical model. *Journal of Homosexuality*, 4, 219–235.

Diamond, L. M. (2012). The desire disorder in research on sexual orientation in women: Contributions of dynamical systems theory. *Archives of Sexual Behavior*, 41, 73–83

Lake, Alison (2018) Extract from unpublished dissertation: *Dear Bob, I love Brenda and It May Impact My Mental Health* [email] (personal communication).

Myers, E.J., & Raup, L.J. (1989). The empty nest syndrome: Myth or reality? *Journal of Counseling & Development*, 68(2), 180–183.

Zanzal, Anne-Marie (2019). *Coming Out Later in Life: A Personal Journey*. After Ellen website https://afterellen.com/coming-out-later-in-life-a-personal-journey/.

Chapter 7

A Gay Son and His Dying Straight Dad*

An Account of Ambiguous Loss and the Embodiment of Homophobia

Paul V. Ricketts

Introduction

As personal embodied experiences can be illuminative, this chapter is written from my personal voice and embodied experience as a gay man on the loss of my father. Auto-phenomenography is a method predominantly based on understanding of embodied experiences produced through autobiographical writing (Kincel, 2017). While auto-ethnography may be a more common term, I include auto-phenomenography because my autobiographical writing has also been about understanding important and essential embodied experiences, part of which is the embodiment of homophobia. I include auto-ethnographic because my story links to the wider socio-political-cultural field.

'Ambiguous Loss' in Death and Relationship

My father died in April 2018, aged 87, from cancer. The 'double whammy' of loss on top of loss became more usefully understood as 'ambiguous loss'. Pauline Boss (1999) describes this as either "people being perceived by their families as physically absent but psychological present" or "physically present but psychologically [and emotionally] absent" (pp. 8/9). As the dying process progressed, my father gradually became more and more physically absent and recognised that we had become psychologically and emotionally absent (increasingly distant) with one another over my lifetime. For me, the dying process was not an emotional time as such and in fact I was glad that I was able to meet his personal care needs and was there overnight before his death. He was, after all, 87 and had had 'a good life'. It was a peaceful, family occasion. It's only sometime afterwards that the realisation of the overall loss/absence began to emerge.

---

* Developmental Somatic Psychotherapy offers "**a template for understanding and working with early psycho-physical blocks** as they emerge in present moments of the adult therapy session" (Frank, 2018).

DOI: 10.4324/9781003335344-7

For instance, I do not remember either of us ever hugging each other – from a little boy onwards. Un-less I've forgotten this. I do remember many instances of him wanting me to be a tough little boy. One example, is a photograph of me being balanced (rather precariously for me) on top of a wall of a bridge that ran across the River Avon with no hand behind my back for support and reassurance. In taking the photo, my mother could see my distress and asked him to hold me. "He's alright", he said. I was only two or three years old.

As time has progressed, I feel much closer to him and have compassion for him and regret the loss of our relationship, and my part in that. I am beginning to miss him and appreciate just how difficult and challenging it must have been for him to have a gay son. I am also realising the probability of him mourning the loss of relationship with me! I will never really know. As I read this back I notice I feel deep regret and sadness with a deep emptiness in my stomach and there also a sense longing and yearning. I also notice a shrinking of my rib cage and I border on the edge of tears with a tightening of my jaw.

During bereavement counselling at a local hospice, I gained peace of mind through recognising and accepting my rejection of my father, and the possibility of loving him not only for his confidence, self-assuredness and strong work ethic but as a whole person despite his shortcomings. At a retreat, soon after, I worked with the idea of becoming 'the father' along the lines of the "prodigal son" biblical narrative (Nouwen, 1994). This idea prompted me to think about my place/position in the family and the wider field of the community of men in regards to that occupied by my father – a perspective, I would never have considered before. Despite his homophobic rejection of me, it helped me greatly in visiting his grave soon after and apologising for my rejection of him. I still feel deep sadness that I was able to reject him without thinking about the impact that would have had on my father. I can only imagine how he must have felt. But I was also angry, hurt, confused and very alone.

Growing up and since, what I valued and appreciated was my father's work ethic. He came from a poor English family but he was a proud man, always worked hard, and was never out of work and was very much the 'traditional breadwinner'. He also played hard and enjoyed his visits to the pub, but always took my mother out on a Saturday night as we were growing up. He was a 'traditional' family man who was well liked by his many friends in the workplace and also by other married couples. When he was younger, he was renowned for being very protective of his older brother and younger brother, and was not afraid of getting into fights on their behalf. He was quite a personality. He also had three daughters, two older and one younger than myself. He was very much a 'man's man' – heterosexual, homophobic, racist and sexist. And then there was me. There is an interesting take on working class masculinity through a relationship between a gay son and his father (Louis, 2018).

The moment I knew I was somehow different was when my primary school teacher said I was "a bit effeminate" to my mother who replied "I know, I am hoping he will grow out of it". I remember feeling puzzled, feeling very alone and retroflected my feelings, but I know they were expressed outwardly in poor appetite, poor physical development, having a severe stammer and bed wetting. On reflection, it was as though I was expected to understand from an adult perspective how I was meant to be – I hadn't a clue. The expectations were that 'little boys' were at least presumed to be heterosexually masculine and to exhibit those traits in outward behaviour. I was completely puzzled, confused and increasingly withdrew. I felt very alone and had few male friends. I had also started to exhibit sexualised behaviour and not unsurprisingly other boys didn't want any of that.

Throughout adolescence my father showed me how men were expected to light a cigarette, drink a pint of beer, how to stand with legs apart, walk like a man and how to relate to other men and indeed women. He distinctively referred to gay men as being 'poofters', 'nancy boys', 'queers' – advising never to "bend down and pick up the soap in the shower". And my mother said "you'll break many a heart, Paul". As I grew older, it became necessary to hide my emerging same sex attraction by 'acting straight', masculine and having girlfriends.

I have always felt that I have never fitted in the community of '(hetero) men', the wider 'straight world', despite a longing to belong to such a community. Neither have I fitted in with the community of '(homo)men' or the wider LGBTQIA community. I have wondered what it might have been like to be born 'straight'.

Social Class Habitus: Socio-Cultural Situating

The experiences brought up by my father's death, made me aware of the distinct cultural moment we each grew up in, and how this shaped our respective contacting. When we meet with clients with different sexuality/race/class etc. from our own, we meet not only what may be phenomenologically present for the client. Our contacting is also shaped by the situational fields we come from – fields that are themselves riven with systemic oppression.

Elizabeth A. Corpt, in defining Bourdieu's social class "habitus", writes that

> class lives unconsciously in the taste distinctions we make and learn to live within – what he [Bourdieu] calls the 'habitus.' Bourdieu believed that society's ultimate aim was to segregate groups into classes through power distinctions and the promotion of taste distinctions, thus insuring a division of labor suited to meet society's needs.
>
> (Corpt, 2013, p. 60; paraphrasing Bourdieu, 1984; 2013)

This is about segregation through power distinctions and the promotion of and reification of taste distinctions along the lines of the 'haves' and the 'have nots' in economic and cultural capital.

Taste distinctions

> help us determine where we belong, and with whom, and provide us with a sense of who we are, are not, and whom we may or may not become. These distinctions also make demands on us to psychologically define ourselves as we socially declare ourselves.
>
> (Corpt, 2013, p. 61)

It is this sense of belonging that seemed to be a powerful driver for my father as he regularly defended working class values and beliefs. My father hated and despised anything that was not clearly demarcated as being working class – e.g. conservative and liberal politicians, political parties, 'posh' clipped BBC English and artists such as Noel Coward. For me, growing up, there was an element of confusion that lay in my parents coming from two different social class backgrounds. My maternal grandfather, i.e. my father's father-in-law, was a successful small businessman, to whom I looked up to and admired. Over the years, in claiming/reclaiming this aspect of personal identity I am better able to locate my own and my father's experience. It was my grandfather who put a 'roof over our heads'. I believe this was difficult for my father to accept sometimes.

Racism became embedded into the nation's structures of power, culture, education and identity. "People from Africa, the Caribbean and Asia were encouraged by government to come to England. But on arrival here they often faced racism and discrimination, which was not illegal in Britain until 1965" (Historic England, 2020).

The key figure for me in this is my father. He was a proud man, but I remember his shame around wearing wooden clogs as he walked down the cinema isle making an embarrassing noise. I have often wondered whether his shame about being poor contributed to his outward expression of aggression and physical fighting – and it makes sense to me that he would project some of that onto 'a despised other'. For me, I became aware that we were one of the 'have nots' in the most obvious of economic, educational and social terms such as exclusion from social activities. Corpt, acknowledges her own father's racism:

> His solution to his dilemmas of belonging and wanting was to project or split off those aspects of himself that did not measure up to his perception of the norm – those aspects that marked him as "less than." By attributing those aspects to a despised other (italics mine), he was able to keep those parts of himself near but held as the "not-me."
>
> (2013, pp. 61–62)

My father, coming from a poor background whose own family were also openly racist, perhaps even more so, embraced these racist attitudes and brought them home. It was not surprising that as children we picked up these attitudes. More so for me, than my female siblings. I didn't really know any different but wanted to paradoxically 'be like' my father. My father unashamedly used to differentiate us 'white folk' with those black communities (using racist language such as 'darkies', 'nig nogs', etc.) that we drove through on the council house estate on the way to my grandparents' home. Such is the dilemma of loving a racist.

As a traditional man – 'a despised other' included homosexuals. For Fisher et al., "in order to be a *traditional* man [italics mine] a male has to prove constantly that he is not a woman, in the process of which he projects his rejected 'feminine' qualities onto the opposite gender" (p. 18). Even worse, citing the research of Schwarzberg and Rosenberg (1998), regarding homophobia, "fear and hatred of gay men [has] at its core a terror regarding homosexuality's unconscious equation with femaleness and femininity. Male homosexuality, as epitomized by anal penetration, can stir a man's deep fear of emasculation and 'getting fucked')" (Cited by Fisher et al., 2009, p. 19). No wonder my father implored me not to 'bend over' and pick up the soap.

Homophobia

Billy Desmond (2016), argues that "Homophobia is not something that can be addressed only at the intra-psychic or social field of relationships. It is an event at the contact boundary of self/world shared phenomenal field" (p. 50). My understanding of the intra-psychic element is that of the notion of internalised homophobia as an introject that would include self-loathing and hatred. In the social field of relationships, homophobia could be characterised as the highly differentiated relationship between my father and myself in the likelihood he too was shaped by his own era having been born to economically poor white, 'traditional' working class family in 1931. Within that highly differentiated relationship and the same with others there were many homophobic events at the contact boundary of self/world shared phenomenal field. For instance, this was particularly so when I left secondary school and worked as an apprentice electrician. It was a very heterosexual and homophobic environment. When it became known that I was 'different', a welder who was proud Irishman became very violent towards me and threatened me. His mates warned me, "he doesn't like it". I remember getting angry and said something like "like what, what's the IT". But afterwards I became more and more concerned about my safety and left.

A Developmental Perspective

So, how might gestalt understand the embodied experience of growing up gay in a 'straight' world and the lack of field support? According to Allan Singer, "we cannot appreciate the self development and sexual identity formation of any youth without looking first at the social context of the development" (Singer, 2001, p. 181). For "certainly society's [homophobic] attitudes toward sexual orientation and identity … are integrated into the self-structure of the developing subjective person" (Singer, 2001, p. 181, citing Wheeler, 1998b, p. 118). This kind of socio-cultural introjection was at odds with the emerging 'true self' that I felt I needed to suppress. But what is the impact of such introjection of homophobia?

As Singer points out,

> *wherever two males are relating and interacting intimately, we have to remember first of all that both of them are bringing their own history of male socialisation*, which inevitably includes at least some prohibitions against dependency, longing, and need, all of which are tinged or more than tinged with shame.
>
> (cited by Wheeler, 2001, p. 135, original author's italics)

My own experience of shame is rather limited and my energy diverted into my creative adjustment of deflection and denial of my emerging sexuality and a conscious intention to present a heterosexual persona. I remember working very hard to present being straight especially in the workplace referred to above. I had a couple of girlfriends, and one in particular became a sexual relationship. Sadly, I treated her quite badly with a distinct lack of care and attention. Deep down, I knew I was lying. Lying to me and everyone around me.

However, on reflection, my own experience was actually one of trauma. Citing Cassesse (2000), Fisher et al. writes that

> Subject to constant rejection, ridicule, violence, and stigmatization for traditional male code violations, the gay child may accept his culture's view of him as a deviant without gender status among his male peers [italics mine]. Unable to find support for the emotional pain and humiliation of this experience, and typically lacking a secure emotional base within his own family, the gay child's identity is thus 'forged in a traumatic context'.
>
> (Cassesse, 2001c, p. 8, cited by Fisher et al., 2009, p. 24)

That notion of 'deviant without gender status' describes my experience exactly, and I identify most strongly with my identity being forged in trauma context. There was clearly very little if any field support for me. My guess is that people (family, family friends, work colleagues) around me knew that I was different (e.g. effeminate traits), but this was either ignored or tolerated or perhaps even both. But some knew of the trauma but lived in denial or were confused themselves.

Working with clients, what might we do about this kind of deficit?

> For McConville, the concrete manifestations of this developmental pro-
> cess are the adolescents efforts to renegotiate the boundaries of impor-
> tant relationships (disembedding), the growing sensation and awareness
> of a personal and private inner world (interiority), and the implementa-
> tion of these discoveries and accomplishments in the form of new, richer
> behavioural and relational commitments (integration).
>
> (Singer, 2001, p. 180)

However, Singer wishes to point out that "the developmental process of
becoming a self, that is, of disembedding from the family field, discovering
one's interiority, and integrating these discoveries in the form of identity and
relationship, is significantly different for GLB youth" (Singer, 2001, p.181,
author's italics).

It was never possible to renegotiate my relationship with my father, particularly more so with my mother or indeed my sisters and wider family.
Neither was it possible to navigate towards a peer group of likeminded youth,
as one never existed for me. I avoided gay bars as that would have been far too
risky of my parents or rather my father finding out. In regard to my interiority, "the emergent sense of oneself may often be of a self that needs to hide
from contact in order to survive" (Singer, 2001, p. 182). My creative adjustment was almost complete denial and deflection from my emerging awareness
and I presented an outer persona that was 'straight', having girlfriends,
adopting an aggressive attitude, and expressing homophobic views. Thus
there was very little substance to integrate. I had to survive. To do anything
else seemed to me not to be available. I remember being very scared and wondered what might happen to me if I did 'come out'. Of course, I have never
officially done this, although I have sometimes named myself as gay but only
fairly recently. There is a lot of ambiguity still around this for me. It depends
on the field/situation.

Bruce Kenofer points out a limitation of McConville's thesis that "from a
lifespan perspective, there may be a progressive series of disembedding that
occur across the course of a lifetime" (2019, p. 52). While historical approaches
are helpful, "something important may be missing in failing to address what
is unique about the particular developmental challenge [italics mine] that the
client is experiencing at this point in their life" (Kenofer, 2019, p. 57).

The disembedding moments across my lifetime makes a lot of sense to
me. However, my rejection of my father was an ineffectual attempt at disembedding and remained as 'unfinished business' until my bereavement
counselling. For Kenofer goes on to say, citing Robert Kegan's fourth level
of consciousness (Morad, 2017): "this involves the process of disembedding ... from relationships such that one can take a choiceful stance with

regards to one's relationships, rather than being captive and governed by them" (2019, p. 55). However, my particular developmental challenge was at a deeper fundamental level, as it turned out.

My sexual orientation and gender expression had been complicated by what had been named by my gestalt trainers as a 'fragile self process' (Mollon, 1994). Jennifer Mackewn describes "their sense of self, their self organisation, is not stable over time ... [citing Beaumont, 1993, p.85] ... [and] are vulnerable to sudden and severe breakdown of their contact functions in some situations of intimacy or stress" (1997, p.197). Intimacy had been a lifelong source of concern and confusion for me. It was only later in my personal therapy that I realised that my 'fragile self-process' had been caused by a developmentally arresting experience of childhood sexual trauma, which was not prolonged over time but a result of three significant events and relationships.

In addressing this 'particular developmental challenge' to develop "a cohesive sense of self over time" (MacKewn, 1997, p.197), my 'deficit' had somehow been impacted upon not just physically (as I never really felt connected with my legs from a very young age) but also psychologically in aligning with Frank's (2018) linkage of developmental movements to psychological functioning, and over time felt more able to function psychologically (and emotionally) . I felt more (physiologically) connected to what I would describe as my psychological and emotional 'ground'. The impact of this was further developed with some residential training in Relational Living Body Psychotherapy with Julianne Appel-Opper in Berlin. There I found my feet.

Along with the process of integrating these discoveries in the form of identity and relationship (in Singer's words), came a stronger awareness of a distinctive 'cohesive sense of self' that was noticed by my gestalt training group. I would say that this cohesion has been foundational in achieving greater clarity around my identity as a gay man.

What Might This Mean for "How" a Gestalt Therapist Might Support a LGBTQIA Client?

Desmond's advice to therapists is to pay attention to "the pervasiveness of homophobia; the reduction of sexuality to sex; practitioner's responsibility to enquire into their own sexualities; strategies to make shame tolerable; and therapist disclosure" (p. 42). I would add that for me, the reframing of the shame context as a traumatic context as described by Cassese (2001), was both powerful and meaningful. I would never have thought of my experience like that. This perspective could lead into considering working with some clients from a trauma therapy perspective (see Miriam Taylor [2014] and in particular James Kepner [2003]).

It might be prudent to state here that childhood sexual abuse is highly unlikely to be causal of any particular sexual orientation and gender expression but might well be a complication that would need careful consideration in therapy.

This chapter has paid particular attention "to the intersectionality of sex, sexuality, and gender" with "the implicated forces of" such concerns as "race" or rather racism, "age" and in particular social "class" to better understand the "emerging figure of homophobia" (Desmond, 2016, p. 50). However, I would go further and suggest that therapists pay attention to other "aspects of the shared phenomenal field" that could also be "present, lurking for attention" (p. 42). In general terms, following Singer (2001) and Kenofer (2019) the field theoretical perspective might need to include the developmental.

Interestingly, I only have a vague memory of and do not remember explicit work in my personal therapy with my sexual orientation and gender expression with a gestalt psychotherapist for six years. We did talk in general terms about my experience of homophobia from a little boy through to what I remember as a traumatising experience from both staff and students during my time in further education during the 1990s. But I do remember her having what I thought at the time as an 'old-fashioned' understanding of such topics from what she was saying about being aware of being 'fancied' by lesbian colleagues, which suggested to me (although I do not remember specific anecdotal examples) that she had not really explored these issues herself either in training or otherwise. I accept the possibility here that my personal therapy had co-creatively avoided exploration of gender expression and sexual orientation – for could it be that both myself and my therapist had embodied homophobia? I felt 'accepted', nevertheless.

Conclusion

This auto-ethnophenomenographic writing process has provided more ground for my gay orientation. It has enabled me to disembed and reconfigure my relationship with my father. However, I would also add that a significant positive impact on my gay orientation was when I worked for the NHS in my role as a senior health promotion officer with young gay and bisexual men in support of their sexual, emotional, psychological and social health. I was also a therapist in the same dedicated sexual health service working with LGBTQIA clients. During this time I had to work head on with my 'internalised homophobia' as I understood it then, in order to go into secondary schools in a large city in the West Midlands and deliver homophobic bullying workshops to class groups.

Finally, this has also been an exploration of 'how I am embodying homophobia' – a question I had not considered before. Desmond's paper was very useful in this regard in enabling a revaluation of my experience from a field perspective and my part in that co-creation. A good example, would be my part in co-creating and embodying the narrative of homophobia in not just protecting myself from others in the field but also contributing to and even perpetuating homophobia in the field. On that basis alone, this exploration requires more thought and believe I have only just touched the surface herein.

About Paul V. Ricketts, PhD

Paul V. Ricketts, PhD, is a psychotherapeutic counsellor, dance movement psychotherapist (DMP), independent scholar, clinical supervisor and a tutor. He originally trained in humanistic counselling, followed by training in dance movement psychotherapy and is trained in gestalt psychotherapy and development and somatic psychotherapy. He has self-published a revised version of his PhD titled *White Men Don't Dance* ... and has a chapter titled "Configuring the personal/professional self" published in *Learning as a Creative and Developmental Process in Higher Education* edited by Judie Taylor and Clive Holmwood. He was involved in the training of students on the MA in DMP programme and the Creative Expressive Therapy (CET) programme at Derby University. Currently, he is currently involved in the training of therapeutic and psychotherapy counsellors and guides students on body process and movement. His extensive annual CPD involves the Sacred Clown and Bata Clown practice.

References

Appel-Opper, J. (2012). Relational living body psychotherapy: From physical resonances to embodied interventions and experiments. In: Young, C. (Ed.), *About Relational Body Psychotherapy*. Body Psychotherapy Publications. Stow, Galashiels.

Bennett, J. L. (2010). 'Inocencia': case study of a transgender woman without gender dysphoria preparing for gender reassignment surgery. *British Gestalt Journal*, Vol. 19 No. 2, pp. 16–27.

Boss, P. (1999). *Ambiguous Loss: Learning to Live with Unresolved Grief*. Harvard University Press. London.

Bourdieu, P. (1984). *Distinction: A Social Critique of the Judgement of Taste*. Routledge. London.

Cassese, J. (Ed.). (2001). *Gay Men and Childhood Sexual Trauma: Integrating the Shattered Self*. Haworth. New York.

Corpt, E. A. (2013). Peasant in the analyst's chair: Reflections, personal and otherwise, on class and the forming of an analytic identity. *International Journal of Psychoanalytic Self Psychology*, Vol. 8 No. 1, pp. 52–69.

Denham-Vaughn, S. & Chidiac, M. A. (2013). SOS: A relational orientation towards social inclusion. *Mental Health and Social Inclusion*, Vol. 17 No. 2, pp. 100–107.

Desmond, B. (2016). Homophobia endures in our time of changing attitudes: A 'field' perspective. *British Gestalt Journal*, Vol. 25, No. 2, pp. 45–52.

Fischer, S. L. (2016). Figuring out the "Real Consequences of Actions": A Gestalt perspective. *Gestalt Review*, Vol. 19 No. 1, pp. 2–6.

Fisher, A. Goodwin, R. with Patton, M. (2009). Men & healing: Theory, research, and practice in working with male survivors of childhood sexual abuse. Available at www.livingwell.org.au/wp-content/uploads/2012/11/Men_and_Healing_2008.pdf. Accessed 7/7/20.

Frank, R. (2018). Center for Somatic Studies: Movement is the root of psychological functioning. Available at https://somaticstudies.com/developmental-somatic-psychotherapy/. Accessed 24/5/18.

Hawley, D. A. (2011). Therapeutic work with gender identity issues: A response from John L. Bennett. *British Gestalt Journal*, Vl. 20 No. 1, pp. 14–20.

Historic England. (2020). The slave trade and abolition. Available at https://historicengland.org.uk/research/inclusive-heritage/another-england/a-brief-history/racism-and-resistance/. Accessed 8/7/20.

Jacques, G. (1998). Homo-erotic horror. *British Gestalt Journal*. Vol. 7 No. 1, pp. 353–461.

Kenofer, B. (2019). Historical vs concurrent approaches to development. *British Gestalt Journal*, Vol. 28, No 2, pp. 50–58.

Kepner, J. (2003). *Healing Tasks: Psychotherapy with Adult Survivors of Childhood Abuse*. Gestalt Press. Cambridge, MA.

Kincel, A. (2017). Embodying collective gestalts: An autophenomenography of culture, masculinity and sexuality in Gestalt Therapy (unpublished PhD thesis). Brighton University. Available at https://research.brighton.ac.uk/en/studentTheses/embodying-collective-gestalts. Accessed 23/6/2020.

Louis, E. (2018). *Who Killed My Father*. Vintage. London.

Mackewn, J. (1997). *Developing Gestalt Counselling: A field Theoretical and Relational Model Of Contemporary Gestalt Counselling and Psychotherapy*. Sage. London.

Mann, D. (2010). *Gestalt Therapy: 100 Key Points and Techniques*. Routledge. London.

Mollon, P. (1994). *The Fragile Self*. Whurr Publishers. London.

Morad, N. (2017). Part 1: How to be an adult – Kegan's theory of adult development. Available at https://medium.com/@NataliMorad/how-to-be-an-adult-kegans-theory-of-adult-development-d63f4311b553. Accessed 26/6/20.

Nouwen, H. (1994). *The Return of the Prodigal Son: A Story of Homecoming*. Darton, Longman and Todd Ltd. London.

Pribram, E. D. & Harding, J. (2002). The power of feeling: Locating emotions in culture. Faculty Works: Communications. 8. Available at https://digitalcommons.molloy.edu/com_fac/8. Accessed 22/7/20.

Rosenblatt, D. (1998). Gestalt and homosexuality: A personal memoir. *British Gestalt Journal*. Vol. 7 No. 1, pp. 8–17.

Singer, A. (1998). Coming out: Adolescence and gay/lesbian/bisexual identity. *British Gestalt Journal*. Vol. 7 No. 1.

Singer, A. (2001). *Coming Out of the Shadows: Supporting the Development of our Gay, Lesbian, and Bisexual Adolescents*. In: Mark McConville and Gordon Wheeler (Eds.), *The Heart of Development*, Vol. 2. Gestalt Press. MA. USA.

Taylor, M. (2014). *Trauma Therapy and Clinical Practice: Neuroscience, Gestalt and the Body*. OUP. Maidenhead.

Totton, N. (December, 2009). Body psychotherapy and social theory. *Body, Movement and Dance in Psychotherapy*, Vol. 4 No. 3, pp. 187–200. Routledge, Oxford.

Unkovich, G. I. (2018). Orienting myself: A gay dance movement psychotherapist's gender experience in training and practice. *Body, Movement and Dance in Psychotherapy*. Vol. 13. No. 3. Routledge, London.

Wheeler, G. (1998a). *Gestalt Reconsidered: A New Approach to Contact and Resistance.* Taylor and Francis. London.

Wheeler, G. (1998b). Towards a gestalt developmental model. *British Gestalt Journal*, Vol. 7 No. 2, pp. 115–125.

Wheeler, G. (2001). *The Self in the Eye of the Father: A Gestalt Perspective on Fathering the Male Adolescent.* The Heart of Development, Vol. 2. Edited by Mark McConville and Gordon Wheeler. Gestalt press: MA. USA.

Williams, R. (1975). *The Long Revolution.* Greenwood. Westport, CT.

Chapter 8

Activism and Therapy

Sanjay Kumar

My decision to go into training as a psychotherapist in London followed soon after I had come out to myself as gay. I was completing my internship at a historic city centre church in Cambridge, UK, and on my way to becoming a Baptist minister to serve in the Church in South India. It was the late nineties.

Psychotherapy was my way out of service in the Church and India without it doing much damage to myself and my family, causing minimum scandal. Psychotherapy was an acceptable career transition for my family and for me, which made leaving Church ministry bearable. My training in psychotherapy itself became a way in which I began to understand and accept myself. While unlearning most of the negative messages I had internalised about being gay, I used my training to write about equality, diversity and inclusion and felt empowered by doing so. So began the activism.

Coming Out

For many of us who are pioneers in our community, being the first to come out and take a stand, to show up, speak up and stand up for who we are, that very act of 'coming out' is an act of activism. Amy Rees-Turyn (2007) writes in the *Journal of Gay and Lesbian Psychotherapy*,

> For LGBT ... the act of coming out or being out is a basic form of activism. In the context of environmental pressures...[to] come out or be out, it is important to acknowledge both the potential for this basic form of activism to reduce prejudice, and the risk individuals may be taking.

For me personally coming out meant the very real risk of public humiliation and excommunication from Church leadership, which in turn meant humiliation for the immediate and extended family. This happened anyway over the years as more and more people from the community got to know my sexuality. My family has over the years bore much ridicule from so-called friends and family.

DOI: 10.4324/9781003335344-8

I chose to be vocal and speak up against homophobia in my community albeit from the safety of being halfway around the world in London with the use of social media. I noticed that members of my community be it school friends, church friends, school teachers, relatives would not publicly comment or show disapproval and judgement, they would always do it on the sly sending direct private messages imploring me to see the error of my ways and that I must fear the judgement of God and always would suffix it by saying they are only looking out for me and reaching out because they 'love me!' For years I wrote back to every single one of them personally explaining how I've reconciled my faith with my sexuality.

Arguably, I am the first openly gay ex-seminarian from the evangelical community in Bangalore, India. Twenty years on, though now I find there are more straight allies in the community, there are less than a handful of Christians who are out and proud living in their communities, and I'm yet to meet a serving seminarian or ordained minister who is out and proud! Most protest by leaving, it's a survival strategy, so did I, this was my protest: "If you can't and/or won't love and accept me for who I am, then I'm not going to stick around and hold space for you nor give you the joy of my company, skills and leadership." The fact that there don't seem to be many seminarians or ordained ministers who are out and proud in a country of 1.3 billion people is indeed for me a sad and disheartening indication of how slow progress has been in this area in India, particularly in the conservative Christian communities.

I haven't come out to my own family about my HIV-positive status, a secret I've kept from them since 2004, although all the while running workshops and support groups in London for those living with the virus. Holding space for others in similar situations as myself has been for me my way of coping. It has provided me a source of comfort, strength and enabling.

An Activist

My activism over the years has involved marching in protests, shouting slogans and waving banners. It has involved participating in pride parades advocating for the legal rights, liberty and equality for gender, sexual and relationship minorities. Activism enabled me to address my own insecurities about being gay and challenge my own conditioning to look down on my sexuality and those of others like me. Speaking out became a channel for looking in and affirming myself. For what I was speaking up for had a direct consequence on my own existence. I also soon began to realise that if I publicly called myself an activist, it often acted as an armour protecting me against homophobia. Being an activist to me conjures up images of a person who is empowered, unafraid, proud, connected with organisations, aware of legal rights. Such a person would feel formidable, resourceful and powerful. I often experienced that homophobes measured their disapproval if I introduced myself as a gay rights activist. Even though most of my family apart from my father, who is sadly now deceased, are still unaccepting of me, now I find they not only measure their words and actions but surely have also begun to respect my convictions and reality.

A Drag Queen

Another form of activism that I've encountered in the queer community and also in my own life is drag. My understanding of doing drag is that it is a particular art form that involves elements of female impersonation, exaggerated, caricatured, curated and enacted as a way of expression, celebration, entertainment and activism. RuPaul, arguably currently the most famous of drag queens in the world, is quoted as saying, "We're all born naked, the rest is drag." RuPaul has in my opinion done a huge amount for visibility and accessibility for the queer movement worldwide. One of RuPaul's ardent fans and one of India's own drag queens, Maya The Drag Queen, has had an amazing journey on the gay scene in Bangalore for seven years. I asked her how her art has been her way of activism and if it has been therapeutic to which she replied,

> I didn't have to go out with placards, me stepping on the stage is my protest against gender constructs, against patriarchy, against people being discriminatory even in the queer community and has been a way of putting the concerns of the queer community out there and it is so good to see how much change has happened. Drag has also provided so much healing for me, Maya has helped drag Alex out of the closet.

I imagine this testimonial is not unique to Alex whose alter ego is Maya The Drag Queen. I would wager that drag indeed has overwhelmingly helped artists cope with their own sexuality, gender expression and their place in society. It is indeed a bold, brave and effective strategy for coping, healing as well as effecting change in society. I can say that from personal experience as I too have an alter ego, a drag persona called Miss Kohinoor Diamond. She has been around since 2004. She is not a traditional drag queen in the sense of performance on stage, she was more a host not just at parties but also panel discussions. She has been someone I've turned to even in private to cope when life became overwhelmingly difficult emotionally and psychologically. When I became Miss Kohinoor Diamond I would feel energised, confident, ecstatic, powerful, complete. She has over the years been a huge source of healing and support to me and has helped me raise awareness and money for many causes.

A Therapist

Activism begins with the self. When one chooses to come to therapy, it is a big bold brave choice to make. Being in therapy is an active choice one makes to engage, to awaken, to challenge, to question, to explore, to emote, to authenticate, to vocalise, to change oneself. Showing the mirror to oneself, sitting with oneself, listening to oneself, paying attention to oneself is a process by which one may bring to the surface deeply hidden trauma, hurt and belief systems which impact the present in negative ways. Addressing these is where activism also begins.

As a psychotherapist working across continents and peoples, genders and sexualities, and in my own therapeutic journey over the years, I've consistently found that it is good to speak out, it is good to give voice to those parts of us that are hurting, ignored, suppressed and even persecuted, both internally and externally, within one's own being, within couples, families, communities and indeed nations.

I look forward to working as a gay psychotherapist back in India now. As I encounter the resistance, cynicism, scepticism, fear and sometimes even derogation of therapy, I remind myself that these same factors often come in the way of activism. Navigating through these hurdles can of course be tiresome, but the rewards are truly exhilarating for all parties concerned when positive evolutionary, sustainable change occurs.

About Sanjay Kumar

Sanjay is an integrative psychotherapist in private practice Positive Therapy Today, a group work facilitator, activist and trainer. He trained at Regents University London and is a registered member of BACP. Sanjay set up and ran London's first ever counselling service for South Asian gay and bi-sexual men through the Naz Project London. Since then, Sanjay has over the past 20 years conducted many therapeutic group workshops, drop-ins, meet ups and retreats through PACE HEALTH, Loving Men, Stretch Festival, Berlin, Easton Mountain, NY and Positive Therapy Today, offering support to gay and bisexual men from various ethnic backgrounds, particularly South Asian men and men living with HIV. He has also worked as a counsellor for the corporate world with Employee Assistance Programmes such as Lifeworks and the Retail Trust. Sanjay is a former seminarian and Biblical scholar and a student of Vipassana Mediation and other Meditative Mindfulness practices including chakra meditation, which he continually incorporates and integrates into his therapeutic practice.

Reference

Rees-Turyn, Amy (2007). Coming Out and Being Out as Activism: Challenges and Opportunities for Mental Health Professionals in Red and Blue States. *Journal of Gay and Lesbian Psychotherapy*. Vol 11, Issue 3–4, 155–172.

Chapter 9

Compulsive Sexual Behaviours
Moving Beyond the Frontiers of Addiction Thinking

Silva Neves

The topic of 'sex addiction' brings a fierce debate amongst professionals. The 'sex addiction' thinking is primarily informed by addiction studies but the science of sexology is largely missing from the literature. I believe we cannot understand the presentation of sexual compulsivity without the knowledge of sexology as it is a crucial part of the phenomenological field of clients presenting with this problem. Although this chapter is not gestalt-specific, I hope I can bring some clarity on the complex clinical issues clients bring to the consulting room, helping gestalt-trained and/or interested readers integrate it in their modality. I believe that the treatment protocol I propose for sexual compulsivity is adaptable to the gestalt theories/methods.

Words Do Matter

The words 'sex addiction' have dominated the clinical field and become a popular term for the public. The 'sex addiction' movement has made a fast growth since the AIDS epidemic of the 1980s, when many people became afraid of sex, particularly promiscuity, with sensational stories and numerous anecdotes. However, the scientific evidence of such pathology simply didn't follow. Many clinicians criticise 'sex addiction' as a moralistic and sex-negative industry (Ley, 2012; Magnanti, 2012; Bering, 2013; Donaghue, 2015).

The word 'addiction' is a popular term used loosely by the general public to mean doing something they enjoy to excess: 'I'm a chocolate addict', 'I'm a Netflix addict', 'I'm a coffee addict'. However, in the clinical setting, 'addiction' has a much stricter definition, according to the DSM-5 (American Psychiatric Association, 2013). Words that therapists adopt are important because they have the power to reduce the enormous shame clients feel, or they can collude with client's perceived defectiveness, causing further psychological harm. Words also shape how we think. If the therapist has a mindset of 'sex addiction', they are likely to be congruent with their thoughts and employ an addiction-focused treatment, despite it not being underpinned by robust evidence-based outcomes.

DOI: 10.4324/9781003335344-9

Addiction

Calling a behaviour an addiction is a disease-oriented thinking as and of itself because the clinical definition of addiction is a pathology. The Diagnostic and Statistical Manual of Mental Disorders (DSM-5) (American Psychiatric Association, 2013) defines addiction within the context of substance use with the specific criteria: (1) impaired control, (2) social impairment, (3) risky use, (4) tolerance and (5) withdrawal.

It is easy to mistake sexual compulsivity for an addiction because clinicians often hear clients complain about their sexual behaviours being 'out of control', *feeling* like an addiction. However, the behaviours we observe on the surface may not reflect the nature of the problems. In a clinical setting, sexual compulsivity does have symptoms of impaired control most of the time. Social impairment is only observed sometimes. Risky use is rare. Tolerance (mistaken for dissociation) and withdrawal have never been clinically evidenced (Prause et al. 2017). Because of the stark lack of evidence, The American Psychiatric Association excludes 'sex addiction' from the DSM-5:

> groups of repetitive behaviors, which some term behavioral addiction, with such subcategories as "sex addiction", "exercise addiction", or "shopping addiction", are not included because at this time there is insufficient peer-reviewed evidence to establish the diagnostic criteria and course descriptions needed to identify these behaviors as mental disorders.
>
> (American Psychiatric Association, 2013, p. 481)

Grubbs et al. (2020) examined the body of research on 'sex addiction' over the past 25 years in an extensive review which found that: 'much of this work is characterized by simplistic methodological designs, a lack of theoretical integration, and an absence of quality measurement'.The validity of the research supporting the notion of 'sex addiction' is indeed questionable.

The International Classification of Diseases (ICD-11, WHO) classified the condition as 'Compulsive Sexual Behaviour Disorder' (CSBD), under the impulse control category, not addiction. The Medical Services Advisory Committee advising WHO with the ICD-11, clearly states: 'materials in the ICD-11 make very clear that CSBD is not intended to be interchangeable with sex addiction, but rather is a substantially different diagnostic framework'.

Impulsivity and Compulsivity

Impulsivity is understood as acting rapidly and without foresight, usually as a response to an urge: 'I crave something sweet, and before I know it I have a piece of chocolate in my mouth.' Impulsivity is associated with a thrill or increased arousal; the thought of the chocolate brings mouth-watering excitement.

Compulsivity alleviates unpleasant emotions, even if that repetitive act brings negative consequences (Berlin and Hollander, 2008). In other words, an impulse is *moving towards* a thrill, and compulsivity is *moving away* from something unpleasant. The impulse of logging on to the sex hook-up app brings the thrill of the possibility of seeing new sexually available people. Scrolling the app for hours in order to avoid feeling lonely may become compulsive if this particular act is the only resource a client has to alleviate the unpleasant feeling of loneliness.

All of us experience poor impulse control once in a while. Think about the times you ate your favourite dessert even though you were already full. It is a myth that having sex for emotional regulation is a problem, just as there is nothing wrong with having comforting food on a bad day. Indeed, our society is quick to unduly pathologise sex. This is partly because people (and therapists) feel uncomfortable around the topic of sex.

The Problems with the 'Sex Addiction' Approach

The typical addiction-thinking primarily focuses on stopping the unwanted behaviour and avoiding 'triggers' without being curious about the clients' experiencing of their erotic world. In 'sex addiction' therapy, avoiding 'triggers' induces fear of the erotic processes that naturally happen when people are faced with sexual stimuli. When we see an attractive body, it is normal to feel sexual desire and arousal, or to have a fantasy about it. In that moment, we make contact with our erotic self, which is a major part of our sense of aliveness, curiosity, wanting, needing, longing, erotic hunger and desires. It is connecting with who we are, not something we do. In this context, the urge is in congruence with the normal flow of the client's experience. Therapists encouraging the avoidance of 'triggers' may actually encourage the disruption of a normal process, which can make sexual compulsivity worse, as described by so many clients complaining of consistent 'relapse'.

Experts in 'sex addiction' highly recommend 12-step fellowship programmes such as Sex Addict Anonymous (SAA) or Sex and Love Addicts Anonymous (SLAA) (Carnes, 2001; Weiss, 2011; Birchard, 2015; Hall, 2019). This is problematic because it encourages clients to enter a sex-negative programme with hidden religiosity (Neves, 2021b). The Sex Addicts Anonymous book (2005), which is entirely anecdotal, teaches its followers that 'sex addiction' is a progressive disease and the main goal is 'sobriety'. Chakrabarti et al. (2002), however, found that masturbatory guilt induced severe depression and erectile dysfunction. Moreover, Chasioti and Binnie (2021) found that the addiction mindset of 'sobriety' and 'relapse' is a major factor for maintaining clients' distress.

Peter (pseudonym) is a cisgender heterosexual man. He is sexually aroused by being submissive within the BDSM context (Bondage and Discipline/

Dominance and Submission/Sadism and Masochism). He derives much sexual pleasure from it. He was told by his girlfriend that it was 'not normal' and she asked him to 'fix himself'. He was worried about it because his kink was his peak turn-on. After a brief search online, he wondered if he was a 'sex addict'. He joined SAA. He was told that he was 'addicted to BDSM', and he now had to stop all sexual activities, all fantasies and to stop masturbating in order to 'reset'. Peter's SAA sponsor confirmed that having BDSM as a primary turn-on was abnormal, but that he could manage his 'disease' by following the 12-steps. Peter felt more shame about his kink than ever before. The more he tried to repress his kink turn-on, the stronger it got. He experienced depression for the first time in his life, and he felt hopeless because he thought he was failing the programme. He feared he would never be 'cured', his girlfriend would leave him for 'someone better' and he would never find love again. Peter started to think about ending his life, but thankfully, he called me first, for a second opinion.

The 12-step SAA or SLAA programmes, so highly recommended by many therapists, have poor evidence-based research, aren't clinically endorsed, ignore the science of sexology and are a potential risk of harm. I challenge 'sex addiction' therapists to re-think their recommendations to such programmes. We, clinicians, must be held accountable for our recommendations and suggestions because we must uphold our ethical pledge: First, Do No Harm.

The Disorder: Compulsive Sexual Behaviour Disorder (CSBD)

The ICD-11's diagnostic criteria are:

> Compulsive sexual behaviour disorder is characterized by a persistent pattern of failure to control intense, repetitive sexual impulses or urges resulting in repetitive sexual behaviour. Symptoms may include repetitive sexual activities becoming a central focus of the person's life to the point of neglecting health and personal care or other interests, activities and responsibilities; numerous unsuccessful efforts to significantly reduce repetitive sexual behaviour; and continued repetitive sexual behaviour despite adverse consequences or deriving little or no satisfaction from it. The pattern of failure to control intense, sexual impulses or urges and resulting repetitive sexual behaviour is manifested over an extended period of time (e.g. 6 months or more), and causes marked distress or significant impairment in personal, family, social, educational, occupational, or other important areas of functioning. Distress that is entirely related to moral judgments and disapproval about sexual impulses, urges, or behaviours is not sufficient to meet this requirement.

The paradox of having these criteria is that it helps clinicians de-pathologise the condition more than it helps diagnosing it because a majority of the clinical population won't meet the criteria in full for the disorder:

1   Most people have some control over their intense sexual urges (otherwise, we would be seeing people having sex all over the place, all the time. For example, they can delay their urge to watch pornography and masturbate long enough until they have a private space to do so).
2   Hiding behaviours from their partners for several months indicate good functional and organisational skills, being in control and aware.
3   Many people never tried to stop their behaviours before getting caught by their partner.
4   Most people derive pleasure from their sexual behaviours, even if they are in breach of their committed relationship agreements. Braun-Harvey and Vigorito (2016) describe clients' experiencing an erotic conflict rather than a disorder.
5   The marked distress reported by most clients is usually related to their sexual shame induced by moral judgements, or facing a separation after the discovery of betrayal, or the disapproval from society, families or religious beliefs.

Rethinking 'Sex Addiction'

Rather than encouraging clients to be erotically avoidant by avoiding 'triggers' and constantly monitoring their behaviours, with the belief that they're 'broken', it is more helpful to do the opposite, to help clients become more erotically aware. Compulsivity thrives in shame, but it does not survive with awareness. Helping clients understand the functions that their sexual compulsivity serve, how it somehow meets a need, how it attempts to resolve underlying disturbances, is crucial to an effective, sex-positive treatment. Equipped with this conceptualisation, therapists do not need to spend time addressing (or correcting) clients' sexual behaviours. Therapists can focus on the core and existential parts of clients, rather than the behaviours themselves, which are only mere symptoms. When clients fully own their erotic selves, without fear, they can re-align their sexual behaviours with their values, their wanting, longing, desires and their sense of aliveness.

Elijah (pseudonym) felt his compulsive use of webcam sex became out of control and impaired his daily life. His *feeling* 'out of control' came from not knowing why he was doing it. The compulsive behaviours helped him move away from unpleasant feelings, but he didn't know what those feelings were. Before looking at what was wrong, I helped Elijah be curious about his here-and-now experiences: his webcam behaviours brought a sense of peace, sexual pleasure, intense excitement, feeling 'in control' because he could connect with his sexuality without anxiety. He then looked at what felt wrong for him: shame because he struggled to feel sexual with his wife; guilt because he assumed that she would feel betrayed if she found out about his webcam behaviours, although there wasn't clarity on their agreed monogamy boundaries. I encouraged Elijah to be curious about his erotic world, non-judgementally. In that space, he was able to identify for himself that the actual problem was that he had a lifelong anxiety of being sexual with partners. The course of our therapy sessions was partly based on addressing what was behind the anxiety, slowly peeling the layers of complexity, rather than staying focused on the symptoms of the webcam sex behaviours. Elijah's genuine curiosity of his phenomenological processes enabled him to become fully aware of his field and to find the meaning that his webcam behaviour was his way to 'treat' his lifelong sexual anxiety. With this awareness, and learning new ways to resolve his sexual anxiety, the webcam sex behaviour naturally stopped. Shame cannot survive in meaning (Brown, 2012). Meaning dilutes compulsivity.

Awareness of the Client's Erotic Mind

I borrow the seminal work of Jack Morin (1995) to help clients explore their erotic mind with the following enquiries:

1   What is your sexual memory peak turn-on?
2   What are the ingredients that make it a peak a turn-on?
3   What is your sexual fantasy peak turn-on?
4   What are the ingredients that make it a peak turn-on?

These turn-ons are as varied as there are human beings on the planet. The client's erotic mind (also called the Erotic Template) can change over time, but this process of enquiries can begin to help clients be in contact with their erotic selves.

The cornerstones of eroticism (Morin, 1995) is another helpful guide for clients:

1   Longing and anticipation
2   Violating prohibition
3   Searching for power
4   Overcoming ambivalence.

Matt, a cisgender gay man, found bareback sex with strangers extremely arousing because his peak turn-on was the anticipation of sexual pleasure, which was enhanced by 'violating prohibition' ('I shouldn't have bareback sex with strangers') and 'overcoming ambivalence' ('I got away with it').

In my work, I identified ten types of Erotic Boosters: (Neves, 2021a)

1   Visual
2   Olfactory
3   Auditory

4   Touch
5   Stress
6   Boredom
7   Emotional
8   Hormonal
9   Fantasy
10 Environment.

Whilst the exploration of the client's Erotic Template is the map, the Erotic Boosters can help clients land in their erotic world on a body-felt level.

Laura (pseudonym), a cisgender heterosexual woman, felt aroused by the fantasy of having sex with her boss (searching for power), which was enhanced by the imagination of that fantasy (visual) and the feeling of being powerfully in control of a man's pleasure (emotional). Laura did not tell her partner about it but enacted that fantasy with other men, without her partner's consent. In that moment, she wasn't in contact with all aspects of her system within her field, because she had not realised she was searching for power nor did she pay attention to the consequence on her relationship and her partner's feelings. In therapy, Laura became aware of her erotic world and what motivated her to meet some specific needs (resolving her childhood wounds of powerlessness faced with her father's rage). She healed her childhood pain in therapy, learnt boundary settings, engaging with her fantasy within the consent of her relationship either through masturbation or role play with her partner. She took the risk of telling her partner about her fantasy so that she could integrate it in her sex life.

The six principles of sexual health (Braun-Harvey & Vigorito, 2016) help clients navigate their sexual behaviours because the principles are not behaviour-focused concerned with how many times someone does what, but they are a guide for clients to assess whether their sexual behaviours are functional based on important values of sexual health.

1   Consent
2   Non-exploitation
3   Protection from HIV, STI and unwanted pregnancies
4   Honesty
5   Shared values
6   Mutual pleasure.

These can serve as a guide of boundary setting and enabling clients consciously modulate their behaviours with making contact with their environment and withdrawal when the need arises. For example, discussing honesty with Laura (honesty with herself first about her Erotic Template, and then sharing with her partner) about her turn-ons was a pivotal moment for her as she had not paid enough attention to it. The topic of non-exploitation is an important one too because clients can be challenged with their non-consensual non-monogamy: cheating on their partner is taking away their right to make an informed decision about their relationship and their own sexual health, therefore exploiting the trust of the relationship.

The Three-Phase Model

Through my clinical work, I have identified a three-phase treatment model (Neves, 2021a).

1　**Phase 1: Regulation**. Awareness of the needs emerging for understanding impulse control. Adding various resources to manage impulse control and emotional regulations.
2　**Phase 2: Reprocessing**. Treating the underlying causes of compulsivity. Finding the origins of the need – some are childhood needs that hadn't been met. Some are post-trauma stress symptoms. Some are acute chronic stress in the here-and-now.
3　**Phase 3: Reconstruction**. Understanding the healing as growth. This phase is an existential one when clients can begin to see their entire life story into a narrative that makes sense to them, and learn how to stay in touch with their ongoing processes, including their erotic world, the connection with themselves, others and the world. This phase consolidates full awareness.

Tim (pseudonym) was a 35-year-old cisgender gay man in a monogamous relationship but couldn't stop cheating. He agreed to be in a monogamous relationship because he thought it was the thing to do to be 'a good gay man', yet his erotic template pointed him towards polyamorous sexual needs, which he thought of as 'bad gay'. Through his therapy he understood that he disowned a major part of himself as he turned his childhood trauma of homophobia back at himself. By slowly allowing himself to make contact with his sexuality, reducing his shame, and resolving the relational disruption of his homophobic past, Tim became more accepting of his polyamorous desires. He started to connect with the Queer community, within which he eventually felt a great sense of belonging. In therapy, Tim was able to reorganise the perception of his whole field, with a sex-positive attitude. His sexual compulsivity disappeared because he was then able to make conscious decisions about his sexual behaviours in line with his values and integrity. He shared with his partner that monogamy was not part of his Erotic Template, they parted amicably, and he reported that he stopped struggling with his sexual behaviours. In some other cases, the monogamous partner might sometimes accept polyamory and relationships can survive. The most important piece is not to keep a relationship alive, but to allow each individuals to be in conscious and consensual relationships.

Paul (pseudonym) was a 50 year old cisgender heterosexual man. He spent the last 20 years engaging with sex workers on a weekly basis. His behaviour started soon after he got married. Paul had suffered severe parental neglect and attachment ruptures in his childhood; he did not know how to receive love from his spouse because it felt too unsafe. Through our work together, he began to face the pain of his childhood. Paul and I worked on his childhood trauma. By emotionally understanding that his wife was not an extension of his parents, the need to feel loved in the safety of stranger's arms diluted and he became more aware of the quality of love received from his wife. His needs to see sex workers automatically diluted.

Chemsex

Chemsex is a term coined by David Stuart to describe same-sex sexual behaviours whilst using drugs such as crystal meth and GHB. In chemsex parties, the drugs give their users a great sense of connection with no fears of judgement, increasing their sexual desire, pushing shame away. At that moment, it feels just right (Smith and Tasker, 2018).

Internalised homo-negativity is malignant because it sits deep inside the psyche from the very beginning of gay men's lives, which is the result of growing up in a heteronormative world. It can lodge in the subconscious to such depth that it is undetected, like a silent tumour, and, in the worst cases, can turn to suicidal ideations. Internalised homo-negativity, which speaks the message 'I'm worthless' causes problems in gay men attaching to others and pulls the strings of sexual behaviours. In moments of come-downs, the chemically induced connection turns into projections ('all gay men are sluts'), imperatives ('I should be a nice monogamous gay man') and excuses ('it's not that bad, that's what gay men do').

Luke (pseudonym), a 30 year old cisgender gay man was joining chemsex parties every weekend, it was his time of the week when he felt he could engage with his sexuality without shame, a respite from the everyday stress. However, his chemsex episodes impacted negatively on his week, with terrible come-down symptoms, anxiety and sexual shame. He realised that the drugs gave him an illusion of being connected with other gay men but in fact he was almost always avoiding the pain of feeling 'abnormal' in childhood. By confronting his childhood bullies with chairwork, and learning not to apologise for his existence, he was able to connect with other gay men without drugs thus the pull of chemsex diminishing. One step at a time, Luke processed his childhood trauma and he was much more aware of how to navigate the current heteronormative world whilst looking after himself, being attuned to himself. He empowered himself to make meaningful connections with peers, gained a better sense of himself and learnt how to love and receive love.

Conclusion

Sex-positive psychosexual knowledge offers all the essential tools needed to assess and treat compulsive sexual behaviours successfully and ethically. There are many people struggling with sexual compulsivity in need of a sex-positive, non-addiction thinking psychotherapists. I challenge and encourage clinicians to step beyond the frontiers of the addiction thinking.

About Silva Neves

Silva Neves is a COSRT-accredited and UKCP-registered psychosexual and relationship psychotherapist. He is a Pink Therapy Clinical Associate. Silva works in his Central London private practice and online. He sees individuals and couples presenting with a wide range of sex and relationship issues. He specialises in working with sexual trauma and compulsive sexual behaviours. He works extensively with the GSRD community. Silva is a COSRT-accredited clinical supervisor. He is a Course Director for CICS (Contemporary Institute of Clinical Sexology). He is the author of *Compulsive Sexual Behaviours, A Psycho-Sexual Treatment Guide for Clinicians* (2021, Routledge). He is a member of the editorial board for the leading international journal *Sex and Relationship Therapy*. Silva often contributes to articles on various sex and relationship topics and speaks internationally. Silva featured in the BBC programme *Sex on the Couch*.

References

American Psychiatric Association. (2013). *Diagnostic and Statistical Manual of Mental Health Disorders, Fifth Edition (DSM-5)*. American Psychiatric Association. Arlington, VA.

Bering, J. (2013). *Perv: The Sexual Deviant in all of us*. Penguin Random House UK.

Berlin, H.A. and Hollander, E. (2008). *Understanding the Differences Between Impulsivity and Compulsivity*. Psychiatric Times.

Birchard, T. (2015). *CBT for Compulsive Sexual Behaviour. A Guide for Professionals*. Routledge.

Braun-Harvey, D and Vigorito, A.M. (2016). *Treating Out of Control Sexual Behavior. Rethinking Sex Addiction*. Springer Publishing Company.

Brown, B. (2012). *Daring Greatly: How the Courage to Be Vulnerable Transforms the Way We Live, Love, Parent and Lead*. Portfolio Penguin.

Carnes, P. (2001). *Out of the Shadows, Understanding Sexual Addiction*. Hazelden.

Chakrabarti, N. et al. (2002). Masturbatory guilt leading to severe depression and erectile dysfunction. *Journal of Sex & Marital Therapy*, *28*, 285–287.

Chasioti, D. and Binnie, J. (2021). Exploring the etiological pathways of problematic pornography use in nofap/pornfree rebooting communities: A critical narrative analysis of internet forum data. *Archives of Sexual Behavior*, *50*, 2227–2243. https://doi.org/10.1007/s10508-021-01930-z

Donaghue, C. (2015). *Sex Outside the Lines*. BenBella Books.

Grubbs, J. B. et al. (December 2020). Sexual addiction 25 years on: A systematic and methodological review of empirical literature and an agenda for future research. *Clinical Psychology Review*, *82*, 101925.

Hall, P. (2019). *Understanding and Treating Sex and Pornography Addiction*. Routledge.

ICD-11. (n.d.). *International Classification of Disease*. 11th Revision. World Health Organisation. [Available Online]: https://icd.who.int/en

Ley, D. (2012). *The Myth of Sex Addiction*. Rowman & Littlefield Publishers, Inc.

Magnanti, B. (2012). *The Sex Myth. Why Everything We're Told Is Wrong*. Phoenix.

Morin, J., (1995). *The Erotic Mind*. HarperCollins.

Neves, S. (2021a). *Compulsive Sexual Behaviours. A Psycho-Sexual Treatment Guide for Clinicians*. Routledge.

Neves, S. (2021b). The religious disguise in "sex addiction" therapy. *Sexual and Relationship Therapy*. DOI: 10.1080/14681994.2021.2008344.

Prause, N. et al. (2017). The Lancet. [online]. Available from www.thelancet.com/psychiatry. Vol 4, December 2017.

Sex Addicts Anonymous. (2005). *International Service Organization of SAA, Inc.* Third edition. SAA.

Smith, V. and Tasker, F. (2018). Gay men's chemsex survival stories. *Sexual Health Journal*, 15, 116–122.

Weiss, R. (2011). *Cruise Control. Understanding Sex Addiction in Gay Men*. Gentle Path Press.

Chapter 10

Queering Relationships

Daniel Morrison

Our cultural assumptions about relationships can sometimes be so deep as to be unquestioned. Popular culture has for a long time shown us a one-dimensional perspective of homogenised monogamous heterosexual relationships presented as a norm, and deviation from that norm is often seen as threatening or unethical. I position myself in this as someone brought up in white middle class Britain and want to acknowledge openly that this is my initial position, the point from which I unlearned, and continue to unlearn, my own internalised cultural prejudice. This unlearning began in my thirties, later than many, and led me to understand that different is not wrong. Queer is a word I use for myself as a descriptor, but also as a verb. To queer relationships is to take apart that which we think we know, to challenge what is 'right', to examine cultural norms and choose what feels true.

Ethical non-monogamy – or polyamory (I will use the terms interchangeably) is a subject that is becoming more visible. There's a growing awareness that alternatives to monogamy exist. In this chapter I will examine the concept of ethically non-monogamous relationships, look at some of the assumptions around traditional monogamy and illustrate some case studies of alternative models. The case studies are based on real-life examples but are not direct reports from an individual. A form of relationship diversity is bondage, discipline (or domination), sadism (or submission) and masochism (BDSM) or relationships with a negotiated power dynamic, which may be part of a non-monogamous arrangement or may not.

What Is Monogamy?

Human beings are not naturally monogamous. This is a bold assertion to begin with and not one that is generally acknowledged. Some species of animal are naturally monogamous, although this is a rarity. Geese and lobsters take one mate on reaching sexual maturity and never take another, even if their mate dies. Humans very rarely behave in this way, despite the fact that this is held as a romantic ideal. If we were monogamous in the same way as some other species, we would form a sexual romantic connection with one person in our teenage years, and thereafter it would be impossible to feel

DOI: 10.4324/9781003335344-10

sexually or romantically towards any other person, ever. When monogamy is framed like this, it's easy to see how far removed it is from our usual way of being. Serial monogamy is more accurate for the majority of people, taking one partner at a time during their life, having periods of being single before becoming involved in another monogamous relationship. Still, for many, a successful marriage seems to be one ended by the death of one partner, regardless of how happy or otherwise they were during their marriage.

Monogamy as an ideal, and with our current understanding, is a modern invention. In other cultures and other times, it has not been the generally accepted norm. Having an understanding of relationship diversity is not only necessary for working with ethically non-monogamous white Western clients, but also those from other cultures where polygamy, arranged marriage or other relationship structures are part of the cultural heritage.

The tradition of marriage is rooted in patriarchal structures of ownership. A woman's sexual fidelity to her husband is essential for hereditary wealth to be passed on to a biological heir, and therefore women's sexuality has been heavily policed and any suggestion of infidelity punished. Male infidelity has traditionally been more acceptable, whether openly acknowledged or tacitly understood. Gay sex between men outside marriage has been acceptable in many cultures, and extramarital lesbian sex has often been ignored as non-threatening, or not acknowledged as a possibility and therefore invisible. Our expectation of monogamy is therefore intertwined with patriarchal power structures of ownership, both of property and of women.

None of this is intended to imply that there's anything wrong with monogamy. It's a relationship style that works well for many people, much of the time. It can be an equal partnership between consenting adults that meets the needs of both. The problem with it arises when it's seen as the only viable option, with any deviation being met with disapproval, misunderstanding or outright hostility. Mononormative bias, the assumption that monogamous relationships are the right, proper and natural way of relationships (Ansara, 2020) invalidates other relationship styles and further oppresses already marginalised groups.

In Western society, the vast majority of romantic or sexual relationships portrayed in films, TV, advertising and books have been heterosexual, monogamous and between two cisgender people. They assume an ideal of equal power, sexual and romantic exclusivity, and procreative, reciprocal sex. Many stories told in all forms of media are based on deviations from this and resolutions that either reaffirm the sanctity of such relationships or reward the protagonist who best adheres to these unwritten rules. One or both of the partners break the rules of the relationship by forming other sexual or romantic connections or manipulating the balance of power in some way.

Monogamy is not one homogenised relationship structure with universally agreed rules, although many people entering into a monogamous relationship assume that it is. Each relationship will have different boundaries around acceptable behaviour; these may have been discussed or may not be discovered until one partner crosses a boundary, bringing attention to it. An example could be a couple who have been dating for a short while, where one person was also dating other people during this time. That person didn't think they were 'in a relationship' and therefore exclusively seeing one person, the other feels they have been cheated on. In a long-term established relationship, where are the internal boundaries? Is it acceptable to have sexual feelings about another person, fleeting or more long term? Is it acceptable for one partner to fantasise about sex with another person or to have platonic loving feelings towards a close friend? Does the gender of the close friend affect that? Have these issues been discussed, and if not, could the two people involved have very different expectations or assumptions?

Barriers to understanding about ethically non-monogamy arise from cultural conditioning about self-worth and the responsibility of others for an individual's emotional wellbeing. Taking ownership of one's own inner world, expressing needs clearly, communicating boundaries and navigating the rocky waters of multiple relationships are some reasons why those experienced in alternative relationship dynamics may be more psychologically aware than those who are not. This is not always the case but is offered in opposition to the commonly held view that those in multiple relationships are seeking casual partners without commitment or depth of emotional intimacy.

In a survey carried out by Rosie Wilbry (2017), she found that 4 per cent of people considered a fleeting sexual thought about another person to be cheating, and 4 per cent felt that penetrative sex with someone else was not always cheating. Between these two extremes there was a great deal of variety of opinion on what activities are classed as 'cheating'.

Ethical non-monogamy is not cheating. The key difference is that boundaries are openly discussed, usually on an ongoing basis. There is no one way to practise ethical non-monogamy, as will be shown in some case studies below. Possibly the only universal commonality is that everyone involved knows that they are in a non-monogamous relationship and has agreed boundaries. One of these boundaries might be that they don't want to know details of their partners' other partners, but this is a choice they have made for themselves. It's more usual for all partners to know at least some details about one another, and often to meet and form their own relationships with metamours (see terminology in separate section).

One potential issue with non-monogamy is that people can be viewed as need-fulfilment machines, as pieces to fill a gap in an individual's life or in a relationship. An example might be a heterosexual couple who are seeking a bisexual woman to date both of them, and who have strict rules about the parameters of this relationship – maybe she will be required to have equal feelings for both members of the couple, only have sex with them together, not have any outside relationships and vanish if her presence is a threat to the primary couple. This is sometimes known as 'unicorn hunting' and typically is problematic for the 'unicorn', who has her own needs and desires. A similar issue can arise in monogamous dating, which as a concept can be problematic if it's seen as something like an interview procedure – this is the role that is available in my life, these are the needs that must be met by this person, and if they're unable to fill that role and meet all of those needs there's no place for them in my life. It may be that this is more common in the heterosexual world, where members of the 'opposite sex' are potential partners but rarely close long-term friends if there's no attraction on either side.

Terminology

There are some terms in common use in the world of ethical non-monogamy that might be unfamiliar. Some of these are listed below, but it's important to note that there could be variation in what these terms mean to different people. As illustrated above, we might think we have a culturally shared understanding of 'monogamy' but in fact when we ask an individual what it means in their relationship, there can be variation. In therapy, these terms can be seen as a starting point to open up an exploration of what they mean to this client.

- Open relationship: This is generally a couple who are married or in a long-term relationship who are open to having interactions with other people.
- Hierarchical polyamory: There is a primary relationship that is of higher priority than other, secondary, relationships.
- Veto: A partner in a primary relationship has the right to end their partner's other relationships if they're causing difficulty.
- Egalitarian polyamory: All sexual and romantic relationships are of equal importance and are given equal priority.
- Relationship anarchy: There's no distinction between friendship, romantic and sexual relationships; all are of equal importance.
- Relationship escalator: The narrative of a 'natural' progression of a relationship towards more intimacy and commitment over a period of time.
- Solo polyamory: An individual who has several relationships but chooses not to become entangled in sharing their life with someone else, whose primary commitment might be to their own self-care.
- Aromantic: A person who doesn't experience romantic feelings, the dizzy falling in love feeling of new relationship energy.
- Asexual: A person who doesn't feel a desire for sexual interaction with another person.
- Metamour: Two people who are involved in a relationship with the same person are metamours.
- Compersion: A feeling of joy or happiness when your partner is happy with another of their people.

Relationship Diversity in Therapy

Those in non-traditional relationships may face barriers in therapy due to the assumptions of the therapist, fear of judgement or shame. Gestalt therapists are well placed to support clients in this situation if they have examined their own cultural conditioning around healthy relationships. As is often the case, the key to effective therapy is the therapist's ability to be with the client in their experience of the world and our assumptions can interfere with that. It's the personal work of therapists to become educated around lifestyles that they don't share, rather than to expect clients to educate them. A good starting point might be a therapist who is able to say that they know what ethical non-monogamy means in general, and the ways in which it works for some people, but not what it means for this individual client. From this point the client can explain and explore their own relationship set-up without feeling the need to justify or describe the whole culture of polyamory.

Ansara (2020) claims that de-contextualised notions of empathy, "treating all people the same," and active listening are inadequate substitutes for the specific knowledge, skills and insights needed to provide appropriate therapeutic care for polyamorous and multi-partnered people.

Clients may present in therapy with unhealthy relationship dynamics, attachment styles, incompatibility, communication issues or any other common difficulty arising in any relationship. This may or may not be connected to the non-monogamous nature of the relationship, which is something to be explored with the client rather than assumed by the therapist. Issues do arise in non-monogamy that require the support of a therapist, and many of these issues are the same as those occurring in monogamous relationships.

Bill, a client, is feeling insecure in his relationship with his wife. She goes regularly for coffee with her male work colleague and talks about him a lot. She's often messaging and has started keeping her phone more private, where before she'd often ask Bill to check something on it for her. If their relationship is monogamous, Bill could be thinking that she might be having an affair, with the subtext that this is an unethical thing for her to do and could lead to the end of their relationship. Bill might be navigating his feelings of insecurity about their relationship and his fear of things changing, distrust and betrayal by his wife, and uncertainty that he might be making it up and being unfair to her. Asking her about her feelings towards her colleague could be seen as an accusation, met with defensiveness and anger or with confession and guilt. If their relationship is polyamorous, asking her is an invitation to open up a conversation about the dynamic. If Bill is not accusing her of wrongdoing because feelings for other people are within the boundaries of their relationship, then she is free to be open and honest in her response. Maybe she has feelings for her colleague that she'd like to explore and is able to reassure Bill that it's not a threat to their relationship. This communication has the potential to be cleaner and clearer, as the issue becomes Bill's need for a sense that he's important to her and that she's committed to him, and her need to explore a new dynamic that's arising. If this is how the situation is framed, both people's needs can be met and Bill's work in therapy is to look at his own internal structures around safety, love and belonging and ask for his wife's support in that. Hers might be to navigate the excitement of new relationship energy without damaging her more established relationship with Bill.

It's easy to see in this situation how the unconscious bias of the therapist who has internalised the culture of monogamy could influence the direction of sessions without meaning to. We all have these internalised biases, including those who practise non-monogamy, so the polyamory-aware therapist may have to notice and challenge this in clients as well as in themselves.

Ethical Non-Monogamy in the LGBTQIA Community

Alternative relationship structures may be more common in the queer community – the line between friend/lover is less distinct when the dating pool and friendship group are potentially the same people with ex-partners frequently staying part of the same group. There can be a fluidity with individuals moving from being friends to being lovers and back to being friends. Even if a relationship is sexually monogamous, there may be close and loving friendships with ex-lovers or friends who have engaged in casual sex in the past. In queer friendship groups where polyamory is the norm, there can be a complex network of connection, which leads to a multi-faceted, deep and loving support network. This may be a beautifully tangled community where individuals find belonging within a close tribe or chosen family. Of course, there may also be ruptures within this network, which can occur in any relationship dynamic.

Alex's experience

> For me, polyamory is a part of my social network. In my friendship group there are all sorts of complicated dynamics, but it works for us. I might go for a night out with ten people, and they'll all be partners, ex-partners or partners of each other. It's a tangled polycule with a web of intimacy and connection, and I love it. It's hard to keep up with who's seeing who, and sometimes there are ruptures when people have big emotional stuff going on. As a group we're pretty good at managing that and staying in communication. Last night some people came round to have dinner and watch a film – my new girlfriend Chloe, her live-in long-term partner Sasha, my ex Emmie who also used to be in a relationship with Chloe, Emmie's partner Alice who I had a thing with a few months ago and Maz who's asexual but likes cuddles and co-sleeping, and has snuggly intimacy with all of us at various times. We ended up in a big cuddle puddle to watch the film and it was beautiful.

In our group, queerness is integral to the whole network. Before I came out as queer that kind of thing wasn't possible because it's hard to get away from power dynamics in the heterosexual world. There's a feeling, or there was for me, that men get sex and women give it, so after casual sex with men I often felt somehow depleted. It's hard to explain but I wouldn't have felt comfortable sharing intimacy with lots of men and having them all there at once. Maybe it's my internalised slut shame, or maybe it was that the heterosexual dynamic wasn't right for me. The way things are at the moment, it feels like there's a fundamental equality, which means it's easier to have open conversations. I'm not saying it couldn't work for heterosexual people, I'm sure it does somewhere, but I think there's a whole layer of historical structural inequality, which would need to be unpicked before it could feel right for me.

Ethical Non-Monogamy and Kink

In kink communities, it's common for people to be in multiple relationships with different power dynamics or shared interests. This can be a rich and diverse exploration where different needs are acknowledged and valued without the expectation that two people must match perfectly in all their desires.

Emma's Experience

I have a girlfriend who I love very much, who meets all parts of me and shares my life in many ways, although we don't live together. Neither of us want that kind of relationship, and we're both single parents so enjoy keeping our separateness in some ways. I also have a Dominant who is also mentoring me, as my primary kink identification is as a Dominant. I'm learning submission and service and finding new parts of myself through that journey. When we play and I'm submissive, I meet my edges and experience having my limits pushed while being held and loved. It's deep and meaningful and also challenging. It's building trust in myself, my ability to honour my boundaries and also trust in my Sir to push me while keeping me safe. My relationship with my girlfriend is very different and meets a different part of me. There isn't an ongoing power exchange in that relationship, although we play with power and kink in sex. I have other play partners where I take a Dominant role, as I need to have expression of that in my life as well.

The only thing that's really difficult is not being able to be open with my friends and family about who and how I love. My girlfriend is publicly my partner, as we're more entangled with kids and our social life. It feels deeply wrong and dishonest when my Sir is visiting, to say he's my friend. I don't have words for the relationships I have with his other boys, but friendship feels wrong when I use it there as well. There's a closeness and love which is betrayed by not having the right words. Even if I was to try to explain my kink-based relationships to people not in that world, I'd have to explain so much else first. People would think it's just about sex, or weird power stuff, subconscious trauma or mental health, or abuse. It's hard to explain that it's all love, and all the same but in different flavours. I'd like to live in world where I could be out as polyamorous and kinky without fear of losing friends or being misunderstood.

Emma speaks about the minority stress often experienced by those in non-monogamous relationships. She feels it's necessary to hide an important part of her life from those close to her. As with many aspects of marginalisation, the difficulty lies not so much in the difference itself as in the reconciling of that difference with the wider world. For Emma, it's natural and easy to love more than one person but this requires her to constantly make choices about how much of her life to share or filter in any given circumstance. She has to balance her desire to be authentic in connections with friends and family against the risk of people making negative judgments about her relationships, and the stigma that accompanies that.

Other Non-Traditional Relationships

Ethical non-monogamy can be a creative solution to resolving conflicts between relationship needs and other life commitments. A traditional relationship structure might not be compatible with the lifestyle a person finds themselves in, or may be disrupted by life events.

Kim's Experience

I call myself solo polyamorous, or a relationship anarchist. I'm a single parent of two boys with additional needs who are home educated, and that's my primary relationship and first commitment. My life is arranged around their needs and that feels good. They stay with their other parent every other weekend and that's when I have time to see people I'm in close connection with. I don't prioritise my relationships based on whether they're sexual or not. I have a circle of close people who I share emotional intimacy with and much of our connection is by video calling and messaging. My kids don't get on well with having visitors, so they don't meet my people. I keep my connections separate from my everyday life and that works for me.

On my weekends off I usually visit one of my connections, and we might have sex or we might not. It depends on how we're both feeling. It's important to me that there's no expectation of that happening. We'll share time, maybe share touch and cuddles, and just hang out. All my connections are people I enjoy spending time with whatever that looks like. I feel more comfortable building that kind of relationship with people who have other more committed relationships, as otherwise I can feel that there's too much expectation and dependence in our connection. It's not that I'm afraid of commitment or mutual support, it's that my capacity for that is filled by my family. I'm available for my connections when I can be, but there are non-negotiable limitations for me on how much I can offer. Because of that, it gives me a sense of safety to know that they have other people to go to. If they're having a difficult time, I need to know they're supported without it being my responsibility.

Many of my close people have been in my life for years and our relationship has shifted and evolved over that time. We may go through phases of being more physically intimate, but the most important thing for me is always the friendship and the emotional connection.

The core of my whole relationship philosophy is honesty. My hard limit is that I won't put myself in a position where I have to be dishonest, or my connections do. That means there are uncomfortable conversations sometimes, and I like to check in often with my connections about their other relationships and how our connection feels to them, and if it's working. Sitting with that discomfort and staying true to what's going on for me, and voicing that, and hearing what my close people say, is difficult sometimes but is so important for me. Learning to navigate that has been a huge part of my personal journey and growth over the last few years.

Often there isn't time for a full-time traditional relationship because of other life commitments. Non-traditional relationships allow for connections to evolve in different ways, for people to feel supported even when they're not able to offer a full-time commitment to a partner.

Neurodiversity and Relationship Diversity

Neurodiverse people may have different needs from relationships or find that traditional relationships are problematic because of widespread expectations. Rather than seeing such people as flawed and unable to sustain connection, what happens if we redesign the relationship structure in a way that works?

Lisa's Experience

I'm autistic and need my own space. I've tried living with other people, and have been in monogamous relationships, but it's never worked for me. I was diagnosed as an adult and up to that point, I thought there was something wrong with me, that I should be able to be like other people and manage a 'proper' relationship. Having a diagnosis and learning about polyamory has helped me to understand and communicate what I need, and feel like it's OK to need that. I'm currently in a relationship with a married couple. My relationship with him tends to be more sexual and with her more romantic and sensual. Their relationship with one another is their primary commitment, but both of them make time to see me and we spend time all together as well. I like knowing that they are a unit and meet each other's needs. I'm not emotionally responsible for them, but we're all supportive of one another. I feel deeply connected to them both and they're an important part of my life, and I'm important to them.

I find dating and small talk difficult, my relationships tend to become emotionally deep quite quickly. The combination of wanting emotional intimacy and clarity on what our relationship is, and needing to spend time alone and be in control of my own life, means that it can be hard to find someone who fits with me in relationships. I know that what most people need wouldn't work for me, so if I was with someone who wanted a more traditional relationship style it would mean either I had to pretend, or they weren't getting what they needed. I want my partners to be happy as well, and the structure we have at the moment works for all of us.

Where to Next?

This is a brief overview of some of the diverse ways people can choose to experience relationships outside the expectation of monogamy. Many excellent books have been written exploring the subject in more depth. An early book was *The Ethical Slut* by Dossie Easton and Janet Hardy. Originally published in 1997 and now in its third edition, this is a thorough and evolving introduction to non-monogamy. *Stepping Off the Relationship Escalator: Uncommon Love and Life*, by Amy Gahran, examines many diverse relationship structures and experiences from an online community. Meg-John Barker's *Rewriting the Rules: An Anti Self-Help Guide to Love, Sex and Relationships* is a friendly invitation to question everything we grew up knowing about how relationships work, and an easy and comprehensive starting point to understanding our cultural assumptions.

It's clear that in looking at relationship diversity, we're encountering a range of spectrums that exist simultaneously and interact in different ways. Nurture needs and sexual needs don't need to be met by the same person. Security and excitement might be found in different places. Coming from a monogamous perspective in the therapy room is heteronormative and ethnocentric, and challenging our beliefs as therapists is an important part of developing cultural competence to work with all clients.

About Daniel Morrison

Daniel Morrison is a psychotherapist in the UK. He specialises in working with clients around gender diversity, ethical nonmonogamy and neurodiversity. He also facilitates workshops on connection and polyvagal theory, supporting participants to learn about their autonomic nervous system and offering practical tools to manage and improve mental health. He is a writer, parent, Queer activist and performer. As a neuroqueer nonbinary trans man he brings his own lived experience to his client work, offering relational and integrative trauma informed therapy.

References

Ansara, G., 2020, Challenging everyday monogamism: Making the paradigm shift from a couple-centric bias to polycule-centred practice in counselling and psychotherapy, *Psychotherapy and Counselling Journal of Australia*, 8(2).

Barker, M. J., 2018, *Rewriting the rules: An anti self-help guide to love, sex and relationships*, Routledge.

Gahran, A., 2017, *Stepping off the relationship escalator: Uncommon love and life, off the escalator enterprises*. Off the Escalator Enterprises LLC.

Hardy, J., and Easton, D., 2017, *The ethical slut: A practical guide to polyamory, open relationships and other freedoms in sex and love*, 3rd edn, Ten Speed Press.

Wilbry, R., 2017, *Is monogamy dead: Rethinking relationships in the 21st century*, Accent Press Ltd.

Chapter 11

LGBTQIA in Rural Ireland*
Lives Creatively Lived

Billy Desmond

One Person's Story

Liam has the look of man who has been weathered by all seasons of the year and all hours of the day, muscular, tanned, with an expressive face that lights up with a smile. The crevices in his face, the toughened skin of his hands and his slow, tentative and heavy gait tell a story that words cannot convey. I sense the density of the atmosphere emerging between us as we meet at the door and walk towards the room. He brushes his hands against the walls, and I sense these are part of his support in this new situation with me.

Liam manages, works and owns a family farm of 300 acres. He knows each stonewall that surrounds the farm that passed down through several genera-tions. He knows it as if it were his lover. He is enraptured by the ever-changing novelty of the unfolding beauty that occurs season through season and year by year.

Liam knows his farmland. He treads it with care and attention, carving out the land's use in his head. He is a person with a deep sense of responsibility to heritage and tradition. It's a family enterprise. His wife, Aoife, whom he met and married in his mid-twenties, and their children Tadgh (16), Owen (14), and Aisling (10), are a part of this. Liam (Catholic), Aoife (Church of Ireland), and the kids educated in non-denominational schools, are known, respected and loved by family and friends in the community. They are involved in local rural life with a variety of local community groups and sport clubs.

Liam and his family are not unique of course. They appear to the world like any other Irish family from a rural and farming background. However, all is not what is seems. Liam is a gay man. Yes, he is married to Aoife, a woman, and has kids. He loves them all and is very much loved by them. He has always known that he is gay. His emotional and sexual desires for men were present from his early sexual awakening as a teenager. He was born on

* Some of the ideas for this chapter were first published in a paper in the Summer 2019 Inside Out Journal / Issue 88.

Please note all names and personal stories used in this article are fictional and any resem-blance to factual people or places is entirely unintended.

DOI: 10.4324/9781003335344-11

the West of Ireland at the time the Stonewall riots occurred in New York City. The Stonewall riots marked the beginning of a gay rights movement. It was a night in June 1969 when the drag queens and gay men and women stood up and fought back against the oppressive policing authorities outside the Stonewall Inn – a pub. However, he could not come out over 30 years ago on this island. Being gay was still a criminal offence. It was illegal until 1993 and it is only in recent years that same-sex couples were given the same rights as heterosexual couples with the Marriage Equality Act, 2015. This fills him with despair and loneliness, as he feels he lives behind a stonewall. This stonewall is one that he can see out through its crevices but is unable to move.

His personal Stonewall is still happening. Liam feels trapped, more so now than ten years ago. Outward expressions of same-sex desire and affection are more visible in the Ireland of today. LGBTQIA (Lesbian, Gay, Bisexual, Trans, Queer, Intersex, Asexual) persons are in public life. Our Taoiseach is a mixed race, gay man in a relationship. LGBTQIA persons live openly in our local communities and are part of our families. He sees how his kids and their friends seem more open about different sexualities. He knows of a close friend's daughter who came out as lesbian and saw how she was welcomed home with her girlfriend. He also recently met a married same-sex female couple that moved to rural Ireland, at a local poetry reading.

He has suffered by living life with his secret. His suffering seems to have become more painful and difficult to endure as he has witnessed the social changes occurring. His mental health has been detrimentally affected over the past decade. He has experienced depression and has had suicidal thoughts. He states that Aoife has experienced the heaviness in their relationship and notices that Liam seems increasingly unreachable. She feels lonely in their relationship but is not able to share her experience with anyone. It seems that Aoife too, feels trapped and is hurting.

Liam and Aoife's situation is not unique. Gay men, lesbian (gay women), bisexual, transgender persons and their partners can feel locked in their family circumstances. People are suffering because they are unable to be honest and open about their sexuality, sexual orientation or gender identity with the people they love and in the communities in which they live. There are few places where support is available for coming out and exploring one's sexuality and gender identity as a parent or older adult, or indeed as a partner of a person who is coming out. In rural communities this is usually more difficult and people often feel shrouded in guilt, stigma and shame. So, how do LGBTQIA older persons and their families in rural Ireland find support to live their lives?

Discovering Creative Ways of Living: a Co-emergent Self that is of the Social-Cultural Context

The expression of identities is of our phenomenal field (Husserl 1999) that has within it the person's 'life space'. Our phenomenal field incarnates our lived body stories over the duration of a life to date. The way we 'self' emerges from and of the interaction of the person and their environment (Perls, Hefferline and Goodman 1951). This 'self' is not static but always in motion. This self is both enduring and momentary. Enduring aspects of identity are integrated and become sedimented as represented in this is 'who I am'. Other dimensions of identity are fluid, ineffable and experienced aesthetically through the lived body as witnessed in this is 'how I am'. As human beings move through the world and the world moves through us (Merleau Ponty 1962), the bodying forth of the self is shaped by a socio-cultural field, a phenomenological field, which presents possibilities for creative living. A fundamental existential given is that of corporeality, as we are always situated bodily in the world and this lived body is lived in relation to the other.

Some people like Liam present as heterosexual and live heteronormative lives when in relation to other people. This involves hiding aspects of their lives to partners, families and friends. They are often burdened by feelings of guilt about their desires. The weight of keeping this secret from a partner can have a detrimental effect on the person and loved ones. Individuals trapped in this situation often live with a feeling of shame and dread that they will be rejected or shunned by their family and community, and there is a fear that their children will be ridiculed at school or may reject them if a parent comes out. This has significant and adverse implications on the mental health and wellbeing of these men and women who live a life as others expect them to. They feel stuck. Enduring aspects of identity are sedimented.

The internet and social media fosters connections as well as potentially increasing isolation in our younger generations. For some older men and women, technology is an invaluable resource that assists them in finding connections with someone of the same sex and gender identity. These may be other persons who are also questioning the intersection of their identities, or are living in similar relational situations. Through the use of online dating apps (e.g. Grindr, Tinder) contact can occur in ways that are discrete. In particular, men are using these apps to connect and meet other men for recreational sex. Men may identify as bisexual, gay or men who have sex with men (MSM). Men visiting a few of the larger cities in Ireland may venture to a gay sauna or sex club where they can meet other men for sex. In many instances it is not just the sex that is a draw for these men. It is through such encounters that an aspect of their same-sex attraction and their emotional desires with men can be affirmed in a safe space without the crippling fear of judgment. Such encounters offer some healing and assuage the suffering and pain they may be experiencing in their daily living. In these aesthetically encounters, vitality is present and thus life is experienced in ways that are enriching, even if ineffable or momentary. In my psychotherapy and clinical supervision practice I have seen how connecting via apps or meeting other persons for social conversation and possibly sex are ways of giving expression to their sexuality. This has kept depression at bay and offers some respite. In some instances such contact has prevented individuals from suicide. Such has been the experience of Liam.

Sometimes, out of recreational sexual encounters an ongoing relationship develops as sex buddies and in some instances emotional and loving relationships form. These are usually lived out in parallel to their primary heterosexual married relationship. Two relationships like twin train tracks that may never meet. All is lived out in secret. People retain secrets and silence themselves out of fear of hurting and being hurt. Of course, this has implications for the other partner and children involved, particularly if the secret is maintained. Eventually, the train track does come to a halt and reality is likely to be revealed. Families discover that the life presented was a sham. This has hurtful and sometimes damaging consequences for all involved. Partners, children and friends may feel deceived.

Liam and Aoife are currently in the midst of this storm. Liam has come out. There is pain and relief in the knowing for them both. It is helping each of them to make sense of their distancing, while acknowledging the love they have for each other that has been changing. However, responsibility lies not with only with the individual or the couple, but with us as psychotherapists and the communities and society we are co-creating, to eradicate the need for hiding. We all have a responsibility to ensure people whose sexuality is not heterosexual or whose lives are not lived within the heteronormative structures of monogamy, opposite sex attraction and fixed gendered roles are not shamed or shunned. In addition, we have a responsibility to consider the supports that may be required for children and teenagers whose parents may have come out or transitioned.

How Can Psychotherapists Self-Organise and Create a Ground to Support Clients Who Present as Non-heteronormative?

We are compelled to a world. We are compelled to meaning-making just as we are hard-wired for connection and relatedness. The exploration of our existence as being-in-the-world is an ontological quest not an epistemological one. We are already submerged in meaning, committed to acts of meaning in our daily living before we distil them into our sensory moment by moment lived experience (Merleau Ponty 1962). Our being-in-the-world, is embedded in an intersubjective world of relationships, a world inscribed with cultural meaning and value judgements. As therapists we cannot truly suspend our judgments and place them to one side (Heidegger 1962). These are inscribed in our bodies and are sensed and felt experientially at a domain of implicit relational knowing. Thus 'bracketing' our assumptions and deeply held beliefs is limited. We have already made meaning. In the context of a heteronormative world I propose that we have an ethical and relational responsibility that requires us to critically examine our own lived bodies immersed in a world by attending to the carnal, fleshy experiences evoked in us as human beings who have desires. The nature of these desires may not fit with the prevailing cultural and social norms, and yet we need to find supports to understand and integrate these bodily.

This world on the island of Ireland is changing, a world where the body was historically negated or objectified. The island has been committed to a continuing and painful examination of its cultural and social beliefs as given, created and inscribed upon our bodies. There is a transitioning from a colonised history where bodies were first dominated by representatives of the British empire and a ruling class. After Irish independence the Catholic church and the negation of the Irish state and its people in taking care of our citizens, particularly women and LGBTQIA persons was omnipresent as documented in explicit legislation and implicit relational and cultural contacting. Unfortunately, some of our citizens were more equal than others and the consequences often led to a feeling of exile and marginalization for LGBTQIA persons. The unitary phenomenon as indicated by the compound word 'Being-in-the-world' (Heidegger 1962) and concept of organism/environment field (Perls, Hefferline and Goodman 1951) suggests that there is no understanding of human beings without an understanding of the world we inhabit and vice-versa. The attitude and wonder of a therapist with a phenomenological attitude of inquiry is "to let that which shows itself be seen from itself in the very way in which is shows itself from itself" (Heidegger 1962, p. 58). Experience and the LGBTQIA experience occurs at the skin boundary between persons and it is 'here' that meaning is revealed. The source of meaning that is already 'there' is revealed in the between 'here and now'. Thus the possibilities of co-creating new meaning can be re-imagined by the co-constructing of a non-heteronormative social-cultural background. This is the ground that human beings seek to expand and explore so that the beauty as revealed in the plurality of human expression is confirmed in the 'now for next' of our person to person encounters.

Pragmatically, with the ongoing changes of Irish society, parents can access supports when their children come out or transition gender. The ground is expanding with new possibilities now more available for those needing support. But how do we continue to create a society where we can support the non-judgemental exploration of changing sexualities, gender identity and coming out for older men, women, non-binary persons in our tightly knit rural communities. How do we offer support for families when one or both parents come out? These and other questions need to be explored by humanistic and integrative psychotherapists. In my experience of training and supervising psychotherapists, issues of sex, gender and sexuality have rarely been examined in depth. The binary constructs of male/female, man/woman and the heteronormative constructs of relationships prevail and thus diminish the possibility for healing and positive change to occur for persons who are questioning gender, sexual orientation and polyamorous or polysexual lives.

When working with persons who may not openly identify as LGBTQIA and are living lives that are seemingly heterosexual but are non-heteronormative, it requires psychotherapists to have the necessary supports to be fully alive in the inter-subjective encounter. Some of the following 'steps' may support this process so clients like Liam are supported and not further shamed or shunned because of their gender, sexual orientation and expression of their sexuality.

Know Yourself

We have an ethical responsibility and duty of care towards our clients and indeed ourselves to critically examine and explore our intersectional identities. This is not a one-off event but an on-going phenomenological inquiry into the lived body, a situated body that alters and changes over the duration of our lives. How aware are you of your gender, sexual orientation and sexuality? What is your experience of your gender, sex, sexuality and what biases, assumptions and beliefs you hold? How do you embody these dimensions of your experience? What embodied responses are evoked for you when you meet someone who does not 'fit' within the heteronormative structures of gender, sexuality and relationship? How curious are you about the expressions of a person's gender and sexuality and how you experience these? Have you explored living in the sex and gender other than that assigned to you? Have you imagined walking hand in hand or kissing a person of the same-sex in public spaces, such as cafe, pubs, at local community gatherings or on the street?

As humanistic and integrative therapists, a lack of awareness and understanding of our gender, sex, sexuality and sexual desires will contribute to the amplification of shame and guilt with clients. It is not what you say or don't say. Your sexuality is present as ground for the contact between you and your LGBTQIA clients, I propose that sexuality is integral to our relationality in the dance we co-create with clients. Dreitzel (2018) goes one step further and posits that our "sexuality supports and strengthens human connectivity" (p. 108).

Your embodied responses will convey your capacity for acceptance and non-judgement to your clients. A minute kinaesthetic movement on hearing the experience of a person as they describe their world of relating that may involve multiple partners, sex-buddies, open relationships etc. will often be a repetition of what the client experiences in the world outside and minimises the opportunity for exploration.

Let's Talk about Sex

Sex positive conversation is necessary. The responsibility rests with us all as psychotherapists, as well as parents, teachers and our local GPs. Goodman (1994) reminds us that "many of my lifelong personal loyalties had sexual beginnings" (p. 111). To co-co-construct a relational field that fosters the possibility for dialogue minimises stigma and shame that has unfortunately been part of our Irish context. Consensual sex with someone whom you have feelings for, whether that is over a lifetime or in a brief encounter fosters physical and psychological well-being. Sex and sex play is a celebration of how we as human beings give expression to our most intimate needs in the world. There are of course risks of STIs and HIV for any person who is sexually active. Exploring how cisgender men and women, trans men and women, and non-binary persons are practicing safe sex or not is part of the work. This is a feature of assessing risk and the capacity of self-care. The availability of PrEP (pre-exposure prophylaxis), a medication that if taken regularly can prevent HIV infection, is allowing men who have sex with men to feel safe, confident and less fearful. It eradicates the risk of transferring the HIV virus between partners. Sex positive exploration supports a healthy response to an integral part of our human expression, where each consenting person in the sexual relationship experiences care and affirmation.

Different Types of Psychological Support: Think Beyond the Individual

Individual psychotherapy can be of tremendous help for individuals to explore their feelings in a safe and confidential environment with the help of an experienced psychotherapist. In the presence of an experienced non-judgemental psychotherapist who understands the beauty and complexity of human sexuality and its expression can support a person to integrate aspects of her/his/their identity that are split off and disowned. Spagnuolo Lobb (2009) reminds us that "[t]he therapeutic relationship represents ... [an] ... opportunity to remake a relational history, restoring certain intentionalities of contact that once bore the seeds of a complete, spontaneous development'" (p. 119). For some individuals gender and sexuality are fluid and not fixed, and change during the course of their lives. And while individual psychotherapy can be a tremendous support, other interventions that incorporate the body stories of lives must be considered so unique creative expressions of the lived body are accepted and confirmed as ground for generative, vibrancy relational contact.

Couple psychotherapy offers a safe environment where both partners who live heteronormative presenting lives (as in the case with Liam and Aoife) can explore the intricacies and intimacies of their relationship without shame being evoked. For any of us in a long-term relationship, you will know that your relationship has changed much over time. In fact, it is as if we are in relationship with different people. We are all changing as human beings due to life events and our hopes and desires for living life authentically emerge as we age. Having a safe and confidential space can support a couple in finding creative and authentic solutions. Indeed it is psychologically healthier for children when parents are clear on their relationship. Some couples choose to stay together with an understanding that one or both will be supported to have safe sexual and loving encounters outside. They live an open relationship. Others choose to find a way of separating.

Openness and honesty is what will be most supportive in the long-term, even if it may be painful initially.

Group psychotherapy for persons exploring sexuality and gender identity or an ongoing weekly group therapy offers clients the opportunities to develop the necessary supports to explore the intersection of sex, gender, sexual orientation and gender roles. Groups are temporary societies. They offer a relational situation where thoughts, feelings and behaviours of a client's life are invited into awareness in a safe and confidential space in the here and now. Over time a client can explore different aspects of him/her/their self in the presence of others and may discover that they are not alone in their explorations.

Foster LGBTQIA Inclusivity

In all local community activities and indeed in our primary and secondary schools, LGBTQIA persons need to be welcomed and affirmed. We as psychotherapists are also members of communities and live in different contexts and are often involved in other local activities. Polster (2021) proposes that community is a support for persons to make sense of their lives as 'community is a substructure of society and provides a more intimate option for people to join their lives together" (p. 72). Consider how you can influence other community members who are often confluent with a heteronormative construct of daily living. When setting up events in Macra na Feirme, ICA, GAA, sports clubs or any community activities, ask the question how is this welcoming to LGBTQIA persons in our community? Is the space safe for people of all genders, sexualities and those questioning to be present without having to hide? How does the language, behaviour and gestures of those organising convey a welcome to all persons? Asking such questions on committees will already make a difference. Questions will start a conversation and create new possibilities. Sometimes, a simple gesture can go a long way. For instance, the inclusion of a welcoming statement or image that invites all people of different sex, gender, sexual orientation, race and ethnicity can be the difference that makes the difference. In so doing you may not only save a life but support members of our communities to live openly and fully.

Conclusion

Over time such considerations as described above will contribute to eradicating the need for secrecy. We know the adverse impact of secrecy and shame irrespective of our sex, gender, sexual orientation or sexuality. The Gestalt psychotherapist who is informed by a relational phenomenological-field orientation is called to live and be available at the contact-boundary in the suffering situation with LGBTQI clients. Such suffering is not inside the person, and not to be resolved by the person in isolation. It is a relational suffering that has the potential to be transformed through a non-heteronormative awareness being available to the psychotherapist. Such awareness when embodied and integrated creates a relational situation that affords the beauty of human expression to be bodying forth with the LGBTQI clients we have the gift of accompanying in our therapy rooms.

So, let's stand proud alongside Liam, Aoife, Tadgh, Owen and Aisling. Let's create a community where we can support them to find their expression as a Rainbow family. These families, like stepfamilies, blended families; trans-cultural and inter-racial families are part of our diversity in this inclusive island of Ireland and beyond.

About Billy Desmond

Billy is a queer cis gender white Irish man, living between the rural West Coast of Ireland and London, England. He works as a Gestalt psychothera-pist, supervisor, and dialogical educator with a particular research interest in embodied ways of knowing in groups and diverse relational dynamics within the LGBTQI (Lesbian, Gay, Bisexual Transgender, Queer, Intersex) commu-nity. He is faculty member at the Gestalt Institute of Ireland, guest faculty at Gestalt training institutes, and a certified trainer of Developmental Somatic Psychotherapy. He is co-chair of the Gender, Sexual and Relationship Diversity Interest Group in IAAGT. He has published journal papers / chapters on group-work, group supervision, experiential ways of knowing in qualitative research, sustainability, spirituality, non-heteronormative rela-tionships, homophobia, gay men, and co-authored a book Introduction to Gestalt (Sage, 2012).

References

Dreitzel, P. (2018). *The Art of Living and the Joy of Life: Development and Maturity in a Changing World*. Siracusa, Italy: Gestalt Therapy Book Series.
Goodman, P. (1994). Being Queer. In T. Stoehr (Ed.) *Crazy Hope and Finite Experience*, pp. 103–118. San Francisco: Jossey-Bas Inc.
Heidegger, M. (1962). *Being and Time*. Oxford, UK: Basil Blackwell.
Husserl, E. (1999). *The Essential Husserl: Basic Writings in Transcendental Phenomenology*. D. Welton (Ed.). Indiana: Indiana University Press.
Merleau-Ponty, M. (1962). *Phenomenology of Perception*. London: Routledge and Kegan Paul.
Perls, F., Hefferline, H., & Goodman, P. (1951). *Gestalt Therapy: Excitement and Growth in the Human Personality*. New York: The Gestalt Journal Press.
Polster, E. (2021). *Enchantment and Gestalt Therapy: Partners in Exploring Life*. London and New York: Routledge.
Spagnuolo Lobb, M. (2009). Cocreation and the Contact Boundary in the Therapeutic Situation. In D. Ullmann. & G. Wheeler (Eds.) *CoCreating the Field: Intention and Practice in the Age of Complexity*, pp.101–132. New York: Routledge, Taylor and Francis Group.

Chapter 12

Gender, Sex, and Relationship Diversity (GSRD) Sensitive Gestalt Psychotherapy

Ayhan Alman

If I strip away the trauma held by my body, I find my essence, my core free from gender and identity. I am all genders and no gender at all at the same time. While I got a glimpse into my essence's nonduality through my spiritual practice and personal therapy, I don't assume this is the reality for everyone. A genderless core makes sense to me, despite my soul feeling comfortable being held by a gendered body. Gender, sex, and relationship diversity (GSRD) involves everyone. We all have thoughts and feeling about who we are, who we love and how we relate, even when we never think about it. In my opinion the absence of GSRD awareness is a sign of privilege and yet it will affect you as a person, a therapist, and those who you work with.

As a queer, Middle Eastern child with Muslim heritage I grew up in countryside Germany all-too familiar with shame about my gender and sexuality. I still feel the occasional waves of inadequacy despite my coming out. My family's need for normality in a foreign culture where we were expected to '*integrate*' always trumped my own need for a happy and healthy life. Living in Germany felt to me like I was driving on the wrong side of the street, and I didn't understand why.

I moved across cities and countries, trying to figure out if I changed the outside whether my inside would also change. The turning point was when I moved to London in 2010. It gave me a pause for the very first time from the stress of not belonging. At the age of 34 years, I sat for the first time in front of a therapist, feeling safe enough to look at my internal chaos.

I became more comfortable within myself and with the help of friends and my most recent therapist I learnt why living in Germany felt so difficult. I now know I am also neurodivergent, which means in simple words I was born with a relational, emotional, and cognitive system that is different from that of most people. Despite being at higher risk of being pathologised, traumatised, and pushed towards the margins, I have found a nurturing ground in London that allowed me to catch up on education and personal growth.

Naturally, I felt drawn towards gestalt psychotherapy when I eventually considered training to become a therapist, due to its creative, experiential, and anti-oppressive nature. In this chapter I will introduce a model for working with GSRD for gestalt practitioners. I will draw the key ingredient for

DOI: 10.4324/9781003335344-12

clinical application from creative indifference (Friedlaender, 1918) which is from my point of view a crucial aspect of gestalt therapy that can make a difference to clients who are struggling with their GSRD.

A Brief History of Gestalt and GSRD

A historical curiosity I found is that in their seminal work Perls et al. (1951/1994) didn't use the word gender a single time, whereas there were 105 mentions of sex and sexuality. When we look at gender binaries (e.g., man/woman, male/female, etc.) we get a clear picture of the gender bias of that time: masculine identifiers (e.g., man, men, male) were mentioned 143 times, whereas feminine identifiers (e.g., woman, women, female) were mentioned 20 times. It's also worth mentioning that Goodman was openly bisexual and did engage in cruising while married to a woman. His female partner didn't object to his activities, but Goodman was still fired from his university job (Taylor, 2004: 511). In summary, even though the seminal work lacks gender awareness – sex, sexuality, and relationships were part of gestalt's DNA.

There are several voices who wrote from a queer male perspective (Singer, 1996, 1998; Jacques, 1998; Rosenblatt, 1998; Levine, 2014; Desmond, 2016; Gillespie; 2017, Kincel, 2021). There are far fewer voices who wrote from a queer female perspective (Huckabay, 1996; O'Shea, 2003; Amendt-Lyon, 2013; Hodgson, 2018). And finally, apart from Kolmannskog (2018) who wrote about a trans group breaking gender norms, there was one case study I could find on transgender experiences written by Bennett (2010) who questions the binary, diagnostic concept of gender dysphoria and a response by Hawley (2011) in the *British Gestalt Journal* (BGJ). I appreciate Bennett's attempt to de-pathologise trans experiences. I concur with Waletich (Chapter 5) who draws out the commonalities between gender dysphoria and trauma and suggests drawing from trauma-informed care.

The Need for a Reliable GSRD-Sensitive Assessment Model

Historically, throughout gestalt's evolution there has been a consistent concern about assessments and its implications. Clarkson asserts diagnosis is reductionist and de-humanising (2004: 27). Joyce and Sills state that historically, diagnosis has often been used 'to depersonalise, objectify or oppress' (2018: 59). Staemmler argues 'exerting one sided power of interpretation' serves the therapist's need for certainty (1997: 42) and Mackewn highlights the risk of treating clients 'more as a case than a person' (1997: 226).

Despite these concerns, Perls et al. were clear that therapists need to 'know in what direction to look' (1951/1994: 228–230). Yontef argues 'ethics and competence' necessitate diagnosis (1991: 397–416) and Melnick and Nevis highlight the benefits of diagnosis (1997: 97–98). When diagnosis is process- and present-based, co-created with the client and considers an 'ever-shifting field' (Mackewn, 1997: 227), it has the potential to help clients and therapists find mutual ground for therapeutic work.

In essence, gestalt's humanistic nature has a lot to offer in terms of depathologising assessment processes. However, the absence of a reliable GSRD-sensitive gestalt assessment model may paradoxically further pathologise GSRD clients, because therapists are at risk to operate from their personal belief system, projections, or worse, from their personal trauma. This can cause harm for clients and therefore it is important we start to integrate existing science and knowledge.

Multilarities and Spectrums

One of the challenges around terminology is that the LGBTQIA community grew over time and there were more and more letters added to make space for various other identities. As our awareness on identities grew, so did our language change. The term gender and sexual diversity was originally coined by sexologist Dominic Davies (2007) and further developed to gender, sexuality, and relationship diversity (GSRD) by Dr M.J. Barker (Davies & Barker, 2015). Davies told me in an email (2022) the latest iteration of the term GSRD changed the word 'Sexuality' to 'Sex' for more inclusivity of intersex lived experiences, because the term sex can mean 'sexuality' and 'biological sex' (Davies & Pink Therapy, 2021).

GSRD guidelines were develop for the British Association for Counselling Psychotherapy (BACP) (Barker, 2017) and the British Psychological Society (BPS) (Richards et al., 2019). It is also important to note, the UK Council for Psychotherapy (UKCP) issued a statement on conversion therapy (UKCP, 2021) to reiterate that gender identity needs to be protected like sexuality. In essence, these guides want to reduce further harm to an already suffering client group.

To develop a simple yet effective model, I have looked at what is already available in gestalt theory. We have Multilarities (Mackewn, 1997) in gestalt which means that our moderations to contact are never black and white but are more nuanced:

retroflection ← expression → violence
egotism ← spontaneity → impulsivity
introjection ← chewing / destruction → spitting out / rejecting
deflection ← focusing / contact → directness / bluntness
projection ← imagination / assumption → owning / literalness
desensitisation ← sensitivity → supersensitivity
confluence ← differentiation / separateness → isolation

Mackewn's Multilarities (1997:107) above tells us that there are grades to moderations to contact. This is exactly what GSRD theory offers. I will break down each GSRD aspect further, but I will start with a disclaimer: As more research emerges and our understanding of GSRD evolves, what follows below is a snapshot in time and may not be conclusive, but rather a summary of key themes. I trust the next generation of gestalt practitioners will advance these concepts once there is more research. I would also like to caution with the words we use. As our consciousness grows, so does our language how we describe experience. It's easily possible that some of these words will be offensive in the near future, because we will have evolved by then. And finally, despite the linear visualisation that will follow, GSRD isn't by all means a linear or rigid spectrum (e.g., the binaries of gay or not gay). Like moderation to contact a GSRD spectrum needs to be considered with nuance within the context of field theory and fluid gestalt formation and destruction processes.

Gender

If we break down gender to its core components there are four key areas that I have adapted from Barker and Iantaffi (2019: 59):

> **Gender Identity** – how a person experiences their inner world and self (see also Almås, Chapter 2):
> man ← trans / nonbinary → woman
> **Gender Role** – a person's interaction with the world based on gender norms:
> hyper masculine ← masculine – neutral – feminine → hyper feminine
> **Gender Expression** – how a person expresses their gender to the world:
> male ← butch – gender nonconforming – effeminate → female
> **Gender Experience** – how a person navigates their world because of their gender:
> hyper masculine ← masculine – neutral – feminine → hyper feminine

Sexuality

If I conceptualise gender as "who am I when I am with myself or with others", then sexuality is "who am I attracted to and what does that says about me". Like gender, sexuality can change over time. The more we become who we are, the more we can love who we love. For some transgender people their sexuality changes during or after transition. For others it remains as before. However, I want to caution that because someone's sexuality can naturally change once the person is more in tune with their self (and sometimes remains fluid indefinitely), it doesn't mean that therapy could or should aim to change their sexuality. This attempt to alter someone's sexuality or gender to conform with biological sex is known as conversion therapy. The practice of conversion therapy is ineffective (American Psychological Association, 2000, 2009; Adelson & American Academy of Child and Adolescent Psychiatry, 2012; Pan American Health Organization, 2012) and harmful (Haldeman, 2002; Shidlo & Schroeder, 2002; Beckstead & Morrow, 2004; Beckstead, 2012). At the time of writing this chapter I found four sub-categories of sexuality useful (adapted from Barker & Iantaffi, 2019):

Sexual Identity – how a person identifies their sexuality
heterosexual ← bisexual / pansexual → homosexual
Sexual Attraction – to how many or whom a person is attracted:
no attraction to others ← one partner & gender → multiple partners & genders
Sexual Roles – what role a person enjoys during sex
submissive ← passive – versatile / switch – active → dominant
Sexual Motivation – the amount of sex a person enjoys
no interest in sex ← low sexual desire – high sexual desire → hypersexual

I'd like to highlight, that heightened sexual behaviour is often misunderstood and mistreated with an addiction model. Neves (2021, see Chapter 9) is an advocate who dismantled why addiction models don't work with sexuality and sex. From my point of view, by separating sexual behaviour from sexual identity, assessments become far less pathologising. Using this fluid and inclusive model applies beyond the LGBTQIA community and encompasses a larger population of people who are struggling with who they are, who they love and how they relate.

Another aspect often causing distress to people is the notion that gender and sexuality are literally interlinked. They are not. Just because a person's gender expression is more ambiguous, neutral or androgyne, it doesn't mean they are either gay or lesbian. Masculine men can be gay; masculine women can be heterosexual; nonbinary people can be attracted to only one gender; trans women can be bisexual. The combinations are endless. We can never assume someone's gender or sexual orientation based on what we see. To give an example, in my gender expression I come across as a man. While I mostly identify with this role that is assigned to me from the outside, my internal world looks different. I feel parts that are masculine, feminine, or gender neutral. What this tells me is that many of the beliefs I hold about gender and what it means is an external social construct that I internalised. From the outside, I appear male and even though my internal world doesn't fully align with this, I am comfortable in my male body.

Relationship

Monogamy centric beliefs have from my point of view biased our understanding of love and relationships (see also Morrison, Chapter 10). Sue Johnson who co-founded emotionally focused therapy (EFT), said in a training video, that according to attachment theory humans engage in serial monogamy (Johnson, n/a), which makes sense if we research heterosexual, cis couples. Unfortunately, this kind of knowledge can lead to unwanted conversion therapy if considered without context: If you believe people are better off in serial monogamy based on science, it is easy to pathologise the person who lives in a consenting non-monogamous (CNM) relationship as someone having commitment issues and shame them without consciously being aware of that. The same applies the other way around: If someone prefers monogamous relationships and is unable to engage in CNM relationships, there is also a risk for conversion therapy if the therapist holds the belief monogamous relationships are less than ideal. Another example of how beliefs can foster conversion therapy is the misconception that BDSM relationships are somewhat linked to trauma (Ansara, 2019). People can move in an out of different relationship preferences and models, whereas some might feel more comfortable to remain in a certain cluster. Relationships are more complex and therefore don't fit into a linear spectrum. Relational binaries appear at first black and white if we consider them on their own.

Relational Binaries (from Barker & Iantaffi, 2019):

together ← → single
monogamous ← → non-monogamous
romantic ← → aromantic
asexual ←→ sexual
partner ←→ friend

However, holding relational binaries as overlapping and interlinked patterns in mind will help to understand that there is more nuance to relationships. If we map these binaries towards types of intimacies, the complexity becomes clearer. Multiple intimacies within different contexts are possible at the same time.

Types of Intimacy (Barker & Iantaffi, 2019: 105):

with self ← with the world around us → with others

Neurodiversity

There appears to be a correlation between transgender people and neurodivergent processes. Anecdotally this is familiar to practitioners who work with transgender clients and there is a growing evidence base to support this link (de Vries et al., 2010). It is beneficial to understand neurodiversity not as pathology but as difference. Attention Deficit and Hyperactivity Disorder (ADHD) and its variations are symptomatically very close to trauma responses. While there is now more awareness about neuro-biological links, it is easily overlooked as a trauma response and vice versa. Understanding that someone's neurology might be different, helps from my point of view to also de-pathologise a person's gender, sexuality, and relationship preferences.

Intersectionality, Race, Ethnicity, Culture, and Abilities

The term intersectionality was originally coined by Crenshaw (2016) to capture overlapping experiences of marginalisation. A black bisexual trans woman might have three intersecting identities where marginalisation can occur. Desmond (2016) argues that homophobia is field phenomenon which also applies from my perspective to lesbophobia, biphobia, transphobia, queer-phobia, intersexphobia, etc. Intersectionality can be conceptualised from a gestalt perspective as multiple overlapping field forces on a person which occur all the same time. Intersectionality involves race, ethnicity, culture, and abilities/disabilities, among other identifying characteristics of a person. In my opinion clinicians have a duty of care to understand the current discourse on race, racism, cultural differences, and ableism in addition to GSRD theory, so that clients are protected from further harm due to lack of education.

The Theory of Creative Indifference in Gestalt

As a practitioner, the most effective way of harm reduction to GSRD clients is in my opinion a simple strategy: adopting a position of creative indifference. My personal interest in creative indifference stems from my challenges during training where my trainers rightly highlighted how I was often missing the client's figure formation and destruction process and was unable to remain creatively indifferent. Wrapped up in my own pain, I often wanted to help the client to feel better about themselves. I needed to learn that my beliefs and values were impacting where my clients went. As such by valuing positivity, I was sometimes worsening the situation where clients felt more inadequate, more shame and more guilt for not being where they thought they needed to be. Having said that, a positive outlook by the therapist is also invaluable for some clients and can be inherently supportive. Creative indifference means to me to disconnect from any outcome and stay with where the client is. It doesn't mean I need to disregard what I believe in. I can still be myself and stay with the client.

In gestalt theory, creative indifference is understood as a *position* (Mackewn, 1997: 66) from which '*polarities co-form*' (Philippson, 2012: XV), 'similar to … *mindfulness*' (Joyce & Sills, 2018: 43). Mann writes it includes '*bracketing* what you imagine might be a way for the client to progress' (2010: 61) and Taylor that it 'underpins the concept of the *horizontal therapeutic relationship*' (2014a: 171). Sonne and Toennesvang argue its objective is to enable increased flexibility in '*gestalt dynamics*' (2015: 73) and therefore the *paradoxical theory of change* (Beisser, 1970) needs to be considered. *Field theory* is also implicated, where 'no part of the total field can be excluded in advance as inherently irrelevant' (Parlett, 1991: 5) as is the related notion of *support*, in line with Jacobs that the therapist cannot know what the client will find supportive (2006: 16). Principles of *existentialism* are also relevant in that gestalt adheres to the principles of *choice, self-responsibility* and *self-actualisation* (Yontef, 1991).

Together this means theories of gestalt formation/destruction, awareness, contact, field theory, support, phenomenology (including horizontalisation and bracketing; Spinelli, 2005), the paradoxical theory of change and polarities amongst others are integral to creative indifference. Creative indifference is an inseparable part of gestalt's holistic model requiring therapists to be open and comfortable sitting with uncertainty. I learnt the most effective way to remain creatively indifferent is to put in an effort and practice and attend supervision and personal therapy so personal challenges don't interfere with clinical work.

Clinical Application

One of the prerequisites for clinical application of creative indifference in GSRD-sensitive therapy is in my opinion that the therapist has attended therapeutically to their own experience of gender, sexuality, and relationship/s, explored their biases as well as educated themselves on the basics of GSRD theory.

Elisa and the Meaning of Femininity

Elisa (pseudonym) is a heterosexual, monogamous, Asian, single woman in her 30s. She sought help from a gestalt therapist to work on her lack of self-esteem. One of her beliefs was that she is not feminine enough and therefore less desirable to men. The therapist suggested that Elisa had some female attributes, like her long hair. He asked her if she would be up for an experiment by wearing a skirt to the next session. Elisa didn't return for the next session.

We all make mistakes as gestalt therapists, and offering this vignette is not about shaming the clinician, but to learn from mistakes that can be avoided with awareness. Here is an idea how the work with Elisa could have unfolded:

ASSESSMENT: Elisa associated her perceived lack of femininity with her single-dom. She thought because she didn't feel feminine enough, she was undesirable by men. Interlinked binaries (as in linking femininity to desirability) are very common when clients explore gender and relationships.

THERAPIST: I'd like to throw in a hypothesis. I might be completely wrong here, but I am wondering if I hear you say because you feel a lack of femininity you are single? And that's because of a belief that men prefer only feminine women?
ELISA: Yes, agree 100 per cent!
EHERAPIST: What do you notice as you hear me reflect that back to you?
ELISA: Mmmh … It makes me sad.

In this exchange between the therapist and Elisa you can see they identified the problem that Elisa is trapped in a polarised gender/relationship bind. Without understanding the field conditions and the context, we cannot just assume that Elisa needs to move towards femininity to find a relationship.

Creative indifference means to stay alongside Elisa as her awareness grows about her subjective experience in the here and now. This can lead to an exploration of why femininity matters to her (because of the influence of media and distortion of beauty standards); how it affects her (feelings of sadness, loneliness, isolation, and inadequacy); and where this belief is originating from (introjected societal forces and norms).

With this vignette I wanted to illustrate that a choice to move towards a side can dysregulate clients, despite the client consenting to an experiment. Encouraging a client to move towards an extreme of a binary perpetuates the notion that we need to be feminine or masculine to be worthy. This is causing so much trouble for so many people, no matter where we are on the gender spectrum.

Chris and Relationship Breakup

Chris is a bisexual trans man who was in an open relationship with his female partner. When his partner decided to break up with him, he was heartbroken and sought help from a cis, hetero therapist. He was very specific that he came for the breakup. As soon as the therapist found out that Chris was trans and bisexual, the therapist's focus became gender and sexuality. In addition, the therapist held firm, negative prejudices about gender and sexuality differences. Chris tried to assert his boundaries several times and left therapy in the middle of the third session extremely agitated and hurt.

Here is an example of how the therapy could have unfolded if the therapist was more GSRD-sensitive:

ASSESSMENT: Chris clearly wants help with his heartache. Neither gender nor sexuality are figural for him and therefore mustn't become the focus of enquiry.

THERAPIST: I hear you are hurting over the breakup. What would be helpful right now?
CHRIS: I don't know what would be helpful. I'm feeling a bit lost.
THERAPIST: We could look at not knowing what you need or at feeling lost. Or maybe there is even something else?

By drawing from phenomenology and horizontalising 'the not knowing', 'feeling lost' and 'else', Chris would have had a choice to express where he wants to go. Creative indifference means to me to strengthen Chris' autonomy and self-agency by trusting that he and his nervous system will know where to go. Of course, as therapists, it's easy to prioritise support and grounding and yet we can never be certain what might be supportive or not (Jacobs, 2006). What we can be quite certain about is that Chris needs a comforting presence of another person who doesn't pathologise him and follows his figure formation and destruction process.

The sad reality is that for many transgender clients, it often feels inherently unsafe to work with therapists who identify with the gender they were assigned at birth (also known as cis therapists), because a simple therapy issue such as a breakup can be quickly misconstrued into a gender and sexuality problem.

Concluding Thoughts

In this chapter I introduced an assessment model based on the concept of multilarities which I applied to GSRD by breaking these down into different spectra. In combination with creative indifference, I believe that gestalt psychotherapy has a lot to offer to help de-pathologise assessment process. I provided two clinical examples of how to work and apply the model. I also showed how the quality of creative indifference unites many key concepts of gestalt and can make a difference to GSRD clients.

The more we are wrapped up in our own challenges in life, the less I believe we therapists can stay with what is going on for our clients. As a result, if we are unaware of our own gender, sexuality, and relationship biases, we are at risk to cause more unnecessary pain to our clients. We cannot ask GSRD clients to educate us when they come for therapy. As therapists, it's our job to know the basic principles of diversity and difference.

Having said all that, it's never a problem to make a mistake or get things wrong. It's OK to struggle with understanding our clients. However, it is not OK to assume that how you live, love and experience life is exactly how everyone else should live, love and experience life.

About Ayhan Alman

Ayhan is a queer psychotherapist with a Muslim, Middle Eastern context, and Western upbringing. He trained as a gestalt psychotherapist at Metanoia Institute in London. Therapeutically, he is interested in how prejudice and bias impacts on the mental health of marginalised communities.

References

Adelson, S. L. and American Academy of Child and Adolescent Psychiatry (AACAP) Committee on Quality Issues (CQI), 2012. Practice parameter on gay, lesbian, or bisexual sexual orientation, gender nonconformity, and gender discordance in children and adolescents. *Journal of the American Academy of Child and Adolescent Psychiatry*. V 51.9, 957–974.

Amendt-Lyon, N., 2013. Relational sexual issues: Love and lust in context. In: Francesetti, G. Gecele, M., Roubal, J., eds. *Gestalt Therapy in Clinical Practice: From Psychopathology to the Aesthetics of Contact*. Istituto di Gestalt HCC Italy, Via S.Sebastiano 38, 96100, Siracusa, Italy. Chapter 28.

American Psychiatric Association (APA) Commission on Psychotherapy by Psychiatrists, 2000. Position statement on therapies focused on attempts to change sexual orientation (reparative or conversion therapies). *American Journal for Psychiatry*. V 157.10, 1719–1721.

American Psychological Association (APA) Task Force on the Appropriate Therapeutic Response to Sexual Orientation, 2009. *Report of the Task Force on the Appropriate Therapeutic Response to Sexual Orientation. American Psychological Association*, Washington, DC.

Ansara, Y. G., 2019. Trauma psychotherapy with people involved in BDSM/kink: Five common misconceptions and five essential clinical skills. *Psychotherapy and Counselling Journal of Australia*. V 7.2, [online].

Barker, M. J., 2017. *Gender, Sexual, and Relationship Diversity (GSRD): Good Practice across the Counselling Professions*. [online] available at: www.bacp.co.uk/media/5877/bacp-gender-sexual-relationship-diversity-gpacp001-april19.pdf [accessed 01/12/2019].

Barker, M.-J. and Iantaffi, A., 2019. *Life Isn't Binary: On Being Both, Beyond and In-between*. [e-book] Jessica Kingsley Publishers, London.

Beisser, A. R., 1970. The paradoxical theory of change. In: J. Fagan and I. Shepherd, eds. *Gestalt Therapy Now*. Science and Behaviour, Palo Alto, CA. 77–80.

Beckstead, A. L., 2012. Can we change sexual orientation?. *Archive of Sexual Behavior*. V 41.1, 121–134.

Beckstead, A. L. and Morrow, S. L., 2004. Mormon clients' experiences of conversion therapy: The need for a new treatment approach. *The Counseling Psychologist*. V 32, 651–690.

Bennett, J. L., 2010. 'Inocencia': case study of a transgender woman without gender dysphoria preparing for gender reassignment surgery. *The British Gestalt Journal*. V 19.2, 16–27.

Clarkson, P., 2004. *Gestalt Counselling in Action. first published 1989*. [e-book] Sage Publication, London.

Crenshaw, K., 2016. *The urgency of intersectionality*. [online] available at: www.ted.com/talks/kimberle_crenshaw_the_urgency_of_intersectionality [accessed 01/08/2017].

Davies, D., 2007. Not in front of the students. *Therapy Today – BACP*. V 18.

Davies, D., 2022. Exchange on GSRD referencing. [email] (Personal communication with Alman, A., 16/05/2022).

Davies, D. and Barker, M. J., 2015. Gender and sexual diversity: Respecting difference. *The Psychotherapist*. V 60, 16–17.

Davies, D. and Pink Therapy, 2021. *What does GSRD mean?* [online] available at: https://pinktherapy.org/gsrd_en/ [accessed 25/05/2022].

Desmond, B., 2016. Homophobia endures in our time of changing attitudes: A 'field' perspective. *The British Gestalt Journal*. V 25.2, 42–52.

de Vries, A. L. C., Noens, I. L. J., and Cohen-Kettenis, P. T. et al., 2010. Autism spectrum disorders in gender dysphoric children and adolescents. *Journal of Autism and Developmental Disorders*. V 40, 930–936.

Friedlaender, S., 1918. *Schöpferische Indifferenz*. Georg Müller Verlag, München.

Gillespie, J., 2017. Pushing into silence: A personal exploration of master/slave sexuality and gestalt. *New Gestalt Voices*. V 2, 78–82.

Haldeman, D. C., 2002. Therapeutic antidotes: Helping gay and bisexual men recover from conversion therapies. *Journal of Gay & Lesbian Psychotherapy*. V 5(3/4), 117–130.

Hawley, D. A., 2011. Therapeutic work with gender identity issues: A response to John L. Bennett. *The British Gestalt Journal.* V 20.1, 14–20.

Hodgson, D., 2018. Reflections on radical respect. *The British Gestalt Journal.* V 27.2, 62–63.

Huckabay, M. A., 1996. Lesbian identity and the context of shame. In: Lee, R. G. and Wheeler, G., eds, *The Voice of Shame.* GestaltPress, Cambridge, MA. Chapter 6.

Jacobs, L., 2006. That which enables: Support as complex and contextually emergent. *The British Gestalt Journal.* V 15.2, 10–19.

Jacques, G., 1998. Homo Erotic Horror. *The British Gestalt Journal.* V 7.1, 18–23.

Johnson, S., n.d. *Dr Sue Johnson's Intensive Course in Emotionally Focused Therapy: Attachment-based Interventions for Couples in Crisis.* [online] available at: https://catalog.pesi.co.uk/sales/pe_001234_eftintensive_011518_organic-85354 [accessed 01/01/2021].

Joyce, P. and Sills, C., 2018. *Skills in Gestalt Counselling & Psychotherapy. [e-book]* 4th ed. Sage Publication, London.

Kincel, A., 2021. *Exploring Masculinity, Sexuality, and Culture in Gestalt Therapy.* Routledge, Oxon.

Kolmannskog, V., 2018. *The Empty Chair: Tales from Gestalt Therapy.* [e-book] Routledge, London.

Levine, A., 2014. Diversifying the ground: Personal, empirical, theoretical, and clinical perspectives on Gestalt contact boundary phenomena in gay men. *The British Gestalt Journal.* V 23.1, 27–34.

Mackewn, J., 1997. *Developing Gestalt Counselling.* [e-book] Sage Publications, London.

Mann, D., 2010. *Gestalt Therapy:100 Key Points and Techniques.* [e-book] Routledge, London.

Melnick, J. and Nevis, S. M., 1997. Diagnosing in the here and now: The experience cycle and DSM-IV. *The British Gestalt Journal.* V 6.2, 97–106.

Neves, S., 2021. *Compulsive Sexual Behaviour: A Psycho-Sexual Treatment Guide for Clinicians.* Routledge, Oxon.

O'Shea, L., 2003. Reflection on Cornell: The erotic field. *The British Gestalt Journal.* V 12.2, 105–110.

Pan American Health Organization (PAHO) (Regional Office of World Health Organization), 2012. *Cures for an Illness that Does Not Exist: Purported Therapies Aimed at Changing Sexual Orientation Lack Medical Justification and are Ethically Unacceptable.* Pan American Health Organization, Washington, DC.

Parlett, M., 1991. Reflections on Field Theory. *The British Gestalt Journal.* V 1.1, 68–91.

Perls, F. S., Hefferline, R. F. and Goodman, P., 1994. *Gestalt Therapy: Excitement and Growth in the Human Personality.* first published 1951. [e-book] The Gestalt Journal Press, Goldsboro.

Philippson, P., 2012. *Gestalt Therapy: Roots and Branches – Collected Papers.* [e-book] Routledge, London.

Richards, C., Gibson, S., Jamieson, R., Lenihan, P., Rimes, K. and Semlyn, J., 2019. *Guidelines for Psychologists Working with Gender, Sexuality and Relationship Diversity.* [online] available at: www.bps.org.uk/sites/www.bps.org.uk/files/Policy/Policy%20-%20Files/Guidelines%20for%20psychologists%20working%20with%20gender%2C%20sexuality%20and%20relationship%20diversity.pdf [accessed 02/01/2020].

Rosenblatt, D., 1998. Gestalt therapy and homosexuality: A personal memoir. *The British Gestalt Journal.* V 7.1, 8–17.

Shidlo, A. and Schroeder, M., 2002. Changing sexual orientation: A consumers' report. *Professional Psychology: Research and Practice.* V 33.2, 249–259.

Singer, A., 1996. Homosexuality and shame: Clinical meditations on the cultural violation of self. In: Lee, R. G. and Wheeler, G, eds, *The Voice of Shame.* GestaltPress, Cambridge, Ma. Chapter 5.

Singer, A., 1998. Coming out: Adolescence and gay/lesbian/bisexual identity. *The British Gestalt Journal.* V 7.1, 24–32.

Sonne, M. and Toennesvang, J., 2015. *Integrative Gestalt Practice: Transforming Our Ways of Working with People. first published in Danish 2013.* [e-book] Karnac Books Ltd, London.

Spinelli, E., 2005. *The Interpreted World: An Introduction to Phenomenological Psychology.* Sage Publications, London.

Staemmler, F.-M., 1997. Cultivated uncertainty: An attitude of gestalt therapists. *The British Gestalt Journal.* V 6.1, 40–48.

Taylor, M., 2014. *Trauma Therapy and Clinical Practice: Neuroscience, Gestalt and the Body.* [e-book] Open University Press, Maidenhead.

Taylor, S., 2004. Paul Goodman. In: De Leon, D. (ed.), *Leaders from the 1960s: A Biographical Sourcebook of American Activism.* Greenwood Press, Westport, CT. 509–514.

UKCP, 2021. *UKCP Statement: Conversion Therapy.* [online] available at: www.psychotherapy.org.uk/news/ukcp-statement-conversion-therapy/ [accessed 01/07/2021].

Yontef, G., 1991. *Awareness, Dialogue & Process: Essays on Gestalt Therapy.* [e-book] The Gestalt Journal Press, Goldsboro.

Chapter 13

"I Assumed That It Was a Man She Was in Love With"*

Heteronormativity and Queer Experimentation in Gestalt Therapy Training

Vikram Kolmannskog

I am a queer-of-colour gestalt therapist, supervisor, and professor at the Norwegian Gestalt Institute University College (NGI). In this chapter I explore heteronormativity among gestalt therapy students and how it can be addressed. This is important for the students themselves, personally, and for the students as future therapists and their clients. While heteronormativity is quite obviously a problem for queer folks, it also limits straight folks, as this chapter will show.

In March 2019, I facilitated an experiment, and did a study in parallel, with a group of students. In the following I first present a conceptual starting point and some existing relevant research and theory. Then I briefly present the experiment and study before I share some observations and reflections that I and the students made in connection with the experiment. I offer this experiment as one that can be used in other therapy training settings to increase awareness on heteronormativity. Hopefully, others' experience and thinking can also be enriched by the particular observations and reflections that came out of it for me and my students. Due to space limitation and my expectation that most readers will be at least somewhat familiar with gestalt, basic gestalt concepts will not be much explained.

Gestalt Therapy, Training and Queerness

'In essential ways, my homosexual needs have made me a nigger' (Goodman 1977:216). These are the words of one of our co-founders Paul Goodman, who was openly bisexual. He continues:

> What makes me a nigger is that it is not taken for granted that my out-going impulse is my right. Then I have the feeling that it is not my street. I don't complain that my passes are not accepted; nobody has a claim to be loved (except small children). But I am degraded for making the passes at all, for being myself.

> (Goodman, 1977:216)

---

* This chapter is based on a Norwegian version published in Norsk Gestalttidsskrift, XVII (2), 2020.

DOI: 10.4324/9781003335344-13

The experience that Goodman describes here – and which I and many queer people will recognise – can be understood in light of heterosexism, heteronormativity, and microaggression. Heterosexism can be defined as "a systematic process of privilege toward heterosexuality relative to homosexuality based on the notion that heterosexuality is normal and ideal" (Dermer, Smith, & Barto, 2010:327). According to McNeill (2013:827), "Heteronormativity promotes the norm of social life as not only heterosexual but also married, monogamous, white, and upper middle class". Microaggressions can be defined as "brief and commonplace daily verbal, behavioral, or environmental indignities, whether intentional or unintentional, that communicate hostile, derogatory, or negative slights and insults toward members of oppressed groups" (Nadal, 2008:23). LGBTQIA people frequently experience microaggressions (Nadal et al., 2011; Nadal, Skolnik, & Wong, 2012; Nadal et al., 2014; Platt & Lenzen, 2013). One type of microaggression is endorsement of heteronormativity by, for example, asking a woman if she has a boyfriend (Sue, 2010). Microaggressions can negatively affect the well-being of LGBTQIA people and cause psychological distress (Balsam et al., 2011; Nadal et al., 2011; Nadal et al., 2014; Robinson & Rubin, 2015; Woodford et al., 2014, 2015; Wright & Wegner, 2012). A single instance may seem trivial – hence 'micro' – but they can have a cumulative effect over time (Sue, 2010). Microaggressions have therefore been compared to mosquito bites (Fusion Comedy, 2016).

As a queer person I sympathise with Goodman, but as a queer-of-colour person I feel mixed about his use of the term 'nigger'. Goodman himself reports that Stokely Carmichael "blandly put us down by saying that we could always conceal our disposition and pass" (Goodman, 1977:216). This resonates with me. I can pass as straight, but I cannot pass as white among other whites. And part of heteronormativity is related to this exact issue: Most people are assumed to be heterosexual, and certain groups or aspects of people are made invisible.

In Norway, homosexuality was decriminalised in 1972. Since 2009 there has been marriage equality. In terms of the law, many LGBTQIA battles have been won and attitudes are changing. According to research, "living conditions for lesbian, gay and bisexual people in Norway in many ways are comparable to those for heterosexuals" (Anderssen & Malterud, 2013:VIII). But, according to the same research, "there are still substantial indications of homonegativity in the population" (Anderssen & Malterud, 2013:VIII). Much heteronormativity and heterosexism – including what the cited study calls 'homonegativity' – is today expressed in more covert ways and is often unconscious and unintentional. Less conscious attitudes can be revealed through tests at www.projectimplicit.net, the webpage of Project Implicit, one of the world's largest psychological experiments and studies. Even I, an openly gay man who comes from a highly educated, progressive family and lives in one of the most gay-friendly countries in the world, received the following conclusion a few years ago when I first tried the test: "Your data suggest a strong automatic preference for Straight People compared to Gay People." This was an eye opener to just how pervasive and internalised heteronormativity and heterosexism still is and how important it is to continue addressing this.

Psychotherapy and psychiatry have a problematic past when it comes to these issues. Homosexuality was a diagnosis – until 1977 in Norway. Up until quite recently, psychoanalytic training institutes in the UK did not accept people who identified as anything but heterosexual, partly because homosexuality could be understood as arrested development in psychoanalytic theory (Newbigin, 2015). In contrast, gestalt therapy has from the start had queer people such as Paul Goodman in prominent positions, and there is nothing in gestalt theory per se that is heterosexist as far as I can see. Quite the opposite, queerness may have influenced gestalt therapy:

> being a nigger seems to inspire me to want a more elementary humanity, wider, less structured, more variegate, and where people pay more attention to one another. That is, my plight has given energy to my anarchism, utopianism, and Gandhianism.
>
> (Goodman, 1977:219)

Arguably, important concepts in gestalt therapy – such as awareness, phenomenology and dialogue – stand in stark contrast to heteronormativity, heterosexism and other forms of oppression. Still, gestalt students and therapists are part of the wider societal field and there will be bias – and much is, as research shows, unconscious and unintentional.

There are several studies on how heteronormativity plays out in the therapy room. A recent Norwegian master's thesis in psychology (Omdal, 2018) involved a literature review on the topic. Omdal (2018:v) writes in the English summary:

> LGB-patients reports [sic] about both positive and negative experiences regarding coming out in therapy. It is important that therapists can meet LGB-patients with openness and acceptance, and avoid both over- and underestimating the importance of their sexual orientation. Some conditions seem to facilitate the process. Clear signs that the therapist has knowledge about, and is open to, sexual minorities is regarded positively. The probability for the patient to come out increases if the therapists manages to not make any assumptions about the patient's sexual behavior and sexual orientation through using gender-neutral language.

There has been little research and thinking about therapy training with regards to gender and sexuality diversity. A gay trainee in a British psychoanalytic institute writes anonymously about his experiences (Anonymous, 2015). He recounts how homosexuality is first raised as a 'perversion' and later as part of a special subject, 'Difference'. While he is grateful for the special subject where homosexuality is raised in a more sensitive manner, he also has some objections and interesting reflections on this:

> This is just to split off anxiety and to communicate that difficulties with sexuality reside exclusively in homosexuals, just as racial problems are the sole reserve of non-whites. Homosexuality belongs to everyone regardless of who they love or how they identify themselves. We have all had a homosexual thought in our lives and if we can't connect with that thought, how can we hope to work in the transference with another?
>
> (p. 9)

A recent American doctoral thesis has researched LGBTQIA microaggressions in counsellor education programs (Bryan, 2017). Results suggest that LGBTQIA students experience a range of microaggressions. One interesting finding is that "neglect of LGBT topics, one frequently mentioned microaggression, meant that they were inadequately prepared to treat LGBT clients, or to manage the experiences of discrimination or bias they encountered in their counseling work" (p. 230). One implication and recommendation is that "Faculty may help students conceive of microaggressions as part of a learning process for all students, and describe how these events will be handled" (p. 233).

I used to identify as a gay man – the G in LGBTQIA – and I still often do. Depending on the situation and context, I today increasingly also identify as queer. This is of relevance to therapy, training, activism, and research. 'Queer scholarship' has been described as 'anti-normative' (Browne & Nash, 2010/2016:7). Rather than being anti, I like to think of my queerness as a questioning, much like a counter-pole to introjection. My position as a sexual minority and oftentimes outsider gives a perspective and distance to certain norms, but I don't think we can live without norms and I don't think it is necessary to react against all norms associated with heterosexuals – we should rather consciously examine them and then choose what to do.

Furthermore, to me being queer involves recognising that identities are fluid, and that construction of categories such as heterosexual and homosexual can be limiting not just for homosexuals but also heterosexuals. As Warner (1993) writes, "The preference for 'queer' represents, among other things, an aggressive impulse of generalization; it rejects a minoritizing logic of toleration or simple political interest-representation in favor of a more thorough resistance to regimes of the normal" (p. xxvi). Browne and Nash (2010/2016:5) write, "Queer theory challenges the normative social ordering of identities and subjectivities along the heterosexual/homosexual binary as well as the privileging of heterosexuality as 'natural' and homosexuality as its deviant and abhorrent 'other'". They go on to say, "While queer scholarship is most often interested in examining the experiences of sexual/gender minorities, some scholars argue for a 'queering' of heterosexual relations as well as including a rigorous analyses of the category of heterosexuality" (Browne & Nash, 2010/2016:5). I believe queerness and queering can be liberating for all, not just sexual and gender minorities. Heterosexuals are also oppressed by heterosexism and heteronormativity. To fit into the category heterosexual they must take great care to be other than homosexual. This is similar to the point made by the gay psychoanalysis trainee (Anonymous, 2015).

I find several similarities between queer theory and gestalt, including the focus on process/fluidity, the revolt against rigid binaries (man/woman, homosexual/heterosexual), playfulness and experimentation. Both queerness and gestalt therapy can also involve a questioning and destabilisation of the binaries of research such as researcher/researched, insider/outsider, theory/ data, research/activism (see also Browne & Nash, 2010/2016).

An Experiment and Study

In March 2019 I did a three-day training with gestalt therapy students at the Norwegian Gestalt Institute. There were 16 students, 12 women and 4 men. Everyone was white except for me. Two were of other European origin, the rest identified as Norwegian. They were in the second half of their third year out of four; the emphasis is then on the therapist role, and most students have their own therapy practice. The topic for these three days of training was 'Sexuality'. I was open from the start about my gay and queer orienta-tion. One student mentioned quite early on that she was lesbian, that she often felt a bit different or alone in the group and was happy to have me as the teacher for three days. On the morning of the second day, I invited the group to do an experiment. My plan, which I didn't reveal, was to increase awareness of, and reflection around, heteronormativity in therapy. I followed a typical gestalt structure of experimentation, observation and reflection. This is in line with the experiential and experimental nature of gestalt ther-apy and pedagogy. It is also similar to action learning and research (Baalen, 2014; Lewin, 1946).

I asked the group to divide into two groups: clients and therapists. I asked the clients to go and wait outside the room. I told the therapists that they would receive a client and work with that person in therapy for 15 minutes. I then went outside to the clients and gave them some instructions. I told them to think of someone they felt some attraction towards, a person of the same gender as themselves or another gender. They should find a therapist and then talk about the attraction and situation. They should do this while trying to not disclose the person's gender, by avoiding gender-specific pronouns, etc. They should notice how this felt and how their therapist responded – whether they revealed assumptions about the gender, whether they mirrored their choice of words, and so forth – and how this response felt to them.

After 15 minutes of therapy, we used the fishbowl structure to share obser-vations and reflections. First the students who had been clients sat in a centre circle for 15 minutes sharing their experiences; the students who had been therapists sat outside and observed them. Then the students who had been therapists sat in the centre for 15 minutes sharing their experiences, the former clients now observing them. I then invited everyone back to the full circle. I asked those who were willing to participate in a study to now write down some experiences on a piece of paper, anonymously, only identifying themselves with gender and age if they were comfortable with that, and then hand in the note to me. To avoid any pressure, I said that people who did not want to participate could just hand in a blank piece paper. Everyone participated. We then continued to share and reflect together as a full group, and now I also prompted them to think theoretically and for us to put theory on the experiences. I then invited those who were willing to write down briefly what they felt was relevant gestalt theory and what they had learnt, and hand in this note to me as well.

In the following section, I present some observations and reflections that I and the students made. This is based on notes I wrote myself during and directly after the training, as well as the notes from the students. The students wrote in Norwegian; I have translated everything to English. I connect these observations and reflections with the existing theory and research that I presented in the preceding section.

Observations and Reflections

The instruction to avoid disclosing the gender of the person they were attracted to, had an effect on many of the students who had been clients. It was mentioned both during the fishbowl sharing and in notes handed in. Woman (33) wrote, "It was very difficult to avoid pronouns in the conversation. I had to search for words and formulations. It led to a 'distancing'." What she describes is not very different from what many of us who are LGBTQIA and queer experience. Perhaps this experiment helped those students who didn't identify as LGBTQIA or queer to empathise more.

Many therapists hadn't expressed any heteronormative assumptions, and this had an important effect on the clients. Man (40) wrote:

> I spoke about attraction to persons outside of my current relationship. The therapist never got to know the gender of these, the persons in or outside the current relationship. It felt good to be met as I was, without anything being added concerning gender.

While we don't know whether this man was LGBTQIA or queer or not, the positive experience seems to be very much in line with other situations when a therapist displays "openness and acceptance" and "manages to not make any assumptions about the patient's sexual behavior and sexual orientation through using gender-neutral language" (Omdal, 2018:V).

However, it also became clear that several clients had experienced their therapist making assumptions. Man (36) wrote:

> I experienced that the therapist concluded (and mistook) the gender of the person that I spoke about and a resistance appeared in me. That remained as a figure for me. I also felt a weak sense of irritation when I felt 'judged' about something the therapist had no way of knowing anything about.

This is in line with several studies on how heteronormativity is present in the therapy room (Omdal, 2018). The experience and response of the client also makes sense in light of research showing that microaggressions can negatively affect the well-being of LGBTQIA people and cause psychological distress (Balsam et al., 2011; Nadal et al., 2011; Nadal et al., 2014; Robinson & Rubin, 2015; Woodford et al., 2014, 2015; Wright & Wegner, 2012).

Already during the first fishbowl with students who had been clients, several talked about their therapist making assumptions and how this had felt. Hearing this, the woman who identified herself as lesbian was clearly emotional, saying how this was such a familiar experience for her, and how much it mattered that everyone here got a sense of it. She also realised that she normally doesn't expect anything else from people and sees it as her responsibility to correct them. Now she was touched by some sense of compassion for herself.

This is in line with existing research showing that LGBTQIA people frequently experience microaggressions (Nadal et al., 2011; Nadal, Skolnik, & Wong, 2012; Nadal et al., 2014; Platt & Lenzen, 2013; Sue, 2010). While the lesbian student didn't mention any negative experiences occurring during training or at the institute, it is worth recalling the research on LGBTQIA microaggressions in counsellor education programmes (Bryan, 2017). In line with this research and recommendations, I sought to make the issue one of relevance to all the students through this experiment, hopefully making everyone better prepared for LGBTQIA and queer clients and to manage experiences of discrimination or bias.

A man – who had often talked about his girlfriend in the group – shared in the fishbowl that he had spoken with his therapist about attraction to a 'colleague' and the therapist had assumed it was a 'she'. He hadn't corrected the therapist. Now he felt a little bit bad for the therapist. He said something along the lines of "I caught the therapist in the trap". Another student in the fishbowl asked him if it had been a pretend act from his side. The man responded that he had experienced attraction to colleagues, "both men and women". He didn't say anything to indicate that he identified as LGBTQIA or queer. This shows how heteronormativity can be limiting for everyone, regardless of whether one identifies as straight or LGBTQIA or queer

(Anonymous, 2015; Browne & Nash, 2010/2016; Warner, 1993). We are many who have felt some attraction to people of various genders at some point (see also Anonymous, 2015).

The experiment, and the clients' sharing in the fishbowl, understandably triggered shame in students who had been therapists and now realised that they had made heteronormative assumptions. When it was their turn to sit in the fishbowl, a woman who had just before heard the student who had been her client share that she had made 'a mistake' and used the wrong pronoun, said that she first reacted with denial and then shame. She said the gender had been irrelevant to her, she was interested in the story and person. Yet, she had – unconsciously – assumed and expressed something about the gender. While gestalt therapy per se can be considered LGBTQIA- and queer-friendly/positive, gestalt students and therapists are part of the wider societal field and there will be bias – and much is, as research shows, unconscious and unintentional.

Soon after this woman's sharing I said something about how heteronormativity forms part of our wider field still (Anderssen & Malterud, 2013). For many the term and concept 'heteronormativity' was completely new. I mentioned an experience with my wonderfully warm and caring general practitioner. He had assumed I talked about a girl, saying 'she', after I mentioned my partner once, and I didn't correct him. I thought it wasn't a big deal, but it was one of many 'mosquito bites', an image used to describe the idea of 'microaggressions' (Fusion Comedy, 2016). Moreover, I mentioned that as a therapist I too have quickly made heteronormative assumptions about clients. In a way I tried to 'help students conceive of microaggressions as part of a learning process for all students', as recommended by Bryan (2017:233). I also wanted to normalise the phenomenon and reduce the shame of the students who had made 'a mistake', clarify that this is a field phenomenon, that it is not that we individually are bad or guilty, and at the same time that we can try to increase our awareness. I recommended Project Implicit to become more aware of bias that we have. I also said that regardless of what happens it can be used in therapy: If you do make 'a mistake', perhaps the client corrects you and this experience can be a useful experience and reflected upon in therapy. If the client doesn't correct you and it later becomes clear that you did make 'a mistake', that too can be useful and reflected upon in therapy. Both situations are after all close to what happens outside of the therapy room. Dialogue, an important gestalt concept, is relevant in any case.

We also spent some time reflecting together as a whole group, including trying to understand what had happened in light of gestalt theory. In the notes handed in, the students highlighted field theory, introjection, confluence, projection, dialogue, and the phenomenological method. One student wrote, " became aware of introjection … How influenced I too am by the field phenomenon in our society – heteronormativity – how easy it is to assume." Another student wrote, "With phenomenology I avoid adding anything to the clients story that is not there." A third student wrote, "Ask questions! Check out! Dialogue." Woman (50) wrote:

> The client described that she was infatuated by a person who was not her husband. The figure was the feeling that she described, a falling in love [...] When the client was in the fishbowl, I understood the task about gender. That I as therapist had said *HE*, I assumed that it was a man she was in love with. That was an awakening! I had not thought about gender at all. It wasn"t important or figure for me [...] A useful experience that I will take with me. How can I assume that she was infatuated/in love with one of the same gender as her husband? [...] I think this is about my own bias and introjection – *PUH*! Instructive!! *Thank you*!

Final Remarks

Arguably, gestalt therapy stands in stark contrast to heterosexism and other forms of oppression. Still, gestalt students and therapists are part of the wider societal field and there will be bias – and much is, as research shows, unconscious and unintentional. In this chapter I have explored heteronormativity among a group of gestalt therapy students in Norway – and how it can be addressed. I presented a simple experiment that I hope will be used by therapy trainers and others to increase awareness on heteronormativity.

The experiment revealed that many students didn't express any heteronormative assumptions. This may be much thanks to our phenomenological approach, an approach that prompts us to not make assumptions but stay as close to the client's reality and truth as possible. However, it also became clear that several had made assumptions. Being told that they had made 'a mistake' understandably triggered shame in students. I believe it is important to normalise the phenomenon and reduce the shame, clarify that heteronormativity is a field phenomenon, that it is not that we individually are bad or guilty. At the same time, I think it is important to communicate that we can try to increase our awareness and become more liberated ourselves and support others in their liberation. Heteronormativity can be limiting for all of us, so a queering of gestalt and the gestalt training is to everyone's benefit.

About Vikram Kolmannskog

Vikram is a queer-of-colour gestalt therapist, supervisor, and professor at the Norwegian Gestalt Institute. He is the author of books of fiction, poetry and non-fiction, including *The Empty Chair: Tales from Gestalt Therapy* (Routledge, 2019).

www.Vikram.no

References

Anderssen, N. & Malterud, K. (eds) (2013). *Seksuell orientering og levekår*. Bergen: Uni Helse/Uni Research AS.

Anonymous (2015). A gay trainee. *New Associations*, Issue 17 Spring 2015. British Psychoanalytic Council.

Baalen, D. (2014) *An introduction to action research: Compendium for 2nd year gestalt therapy students*. Oslo: Norwegian Gestalt Institute.

Balsam, K. F., Molina, Y., Beadnell, B., Simoni, J., & Walters, K. (2011). Measuring multiple minority stress: The LGBT People of Color Microaggressions Scale. *Cultural Diversity and Ethnic Minority Psychology*, *17*(2), pp. 163–174.

Browne, K. & Nash, C. J. (2010/2016) *Queer methods and methodologies: Intersecting queer theories and social science research*. New York: Routledge.

Bryan, S. (2017). *LGBT Microaggressions in Counselor Education Programs. Dissertations*. 3173. Western Michigan University. Available online at https://scholarworks.wmich.edu/dissertations/3173

Dermer, S. B., Smith, S. D., & Barto, K. K. (2010). Identifying and correctly labeling sexual prejudice, discrimination, and oppression. *Journal of Counseling and Development*, *88*(3), pp. 325–331.

Fusion Comedy (2016). How microaggressions are like mosquito bites. YouTube. Available at https://youtu.be/hDd3bzA7450

Goodman, P. (1977). The politics of being queer. In Taylor Stoehr (ed.), *Nature heals: Psychological essays*. New York: Free Life Editions.

Lewin, K. (1946). Action research and minority problems. *Journal of Social Issues*, *34*(6), pp. 34–46.

McNeill, T. (2013). Sex education and the promotion of heteronormativity. *Sexualities*, *16*(7), pp. 826–846.

Nadal, K. L. (2008). Preventing racial, ethnic, gender, sexual minority, disability, and religious microaggressions: Recommendations for promoting positive mental health. *Prevention in Counseling Psychology: Theory, Research, Practice and Training*, *2*, pp. 234–259.

Nadal, K. L., Davidoff, K. C., Davis, L. S., & Wong, Y. (2014). Emotional, behavioral, and cognitive reactions to microaggressions: Transgender perspectives. *Psychology of Sexual Orientation and Gender Diversity*, *1*(1), pp. 72–81.

Nadal, K. L., Issa, M.-A., Leon, J., Meterko, V., Wideman, M., & Wong, Y. (2011). Sexual orientation microaggressions: "Death by a thousand cuts" for lesbian, gay, and bisexual youth. *Journal of LGBT Youth*, *8*(3).

Nadal, K. L., Skolnik, A., & Wong, Y. (2012). Interpersonal and systemic microaggressions toward transgender people: Implications for counseling. *Journal of LGBT Issues in Counseling*, *6*, pp. 55–82.

Newbigin, J. (2015). Rethinking our approach to sexualities. *New Associations*, Issue 17 Spring 2015. British Psychoanalytic Council, pp. 1–2.

Omdal, E. (2018). *Seksuell orientering i terapi – usynlig og antatt heterofil? Å komme ut som homofil, lesbisk og bifil i terapi – en litteraturgjennomgang*. Master Thesis. Bergen: University of Bergen.

Platt, L. F., & Lenzen, A. L. (2013). Sexual orientation microaggressions and the experience of sexual minorities. *Journal of Homosexuality*, *60*(7), pp. 1011–1034.

Robinson, J. L., & Rubin, L. J. (2015). Homonegative microaggressions and posttraumatic stress symptoms. *Journal of Gay & Lesbian Mental Health*, *20*(1), pp. 57–69.

Sue, D. W. (2010). *Microaggressions in everyday life: Race, gender, and sexual orientation.* Hoboken, NJ: John Wiley & Sons.

Warner, M. (1993). Introduction. In Warner, M. (ed.), *Fear of a queer planet: Queer politics and social theory.* Minneapolis: University of Minnesota Press.

Woodford, M. R., Chonody, J. M., Kulick, A., Brennan, D. J., & Renn, K. (2015). The LGBQ microaggressions on campus scale: A scale development and validation study. *Journal of Homosexuality, 62*(12), pp. 1660–1687.

Woodford, M. R., Kulick, A., Sinco, B. R., & Hong, J. S. (2014). Contemporary heterosexism on campus and psychological distress among LGBQ students: The mediating role of self- acceptance. *American Journal of Orthopsychiatry, 84*(5), pp. 519–529.

Wright, A. J., & Wegner, R. T. (2012). Homonegative microaggressions and their impact on LGB individuals: A measure validity study. *Journal of LGBT Issues in Counseling, 6*(1), pp. 34–54.

Index